Dopamine and Neuroendocrine Active Substances

Dopamine and Neuroendocrine Active Substances

Proceedings of the First Symposium of the
European Neuroendocrine Association. Symposium (1st : 1984 :
(E.N.E.A.) Basle, Switzerland, March 4-7, 1984 Basle)

Edited by

Emilio del Pozo
Clinical Research
SANDOZ
Basle, Switzerland

Edward Flückiger
Preclinical Research
SANDOZ
Basle, Switzerland

1985

ACADEMIC PRESS
HARCOURT BRACE JOVANOVICH, PUBLISHERS
LONDON   ORLANDO   SAN DIEGO   NEW YORK
TORONTO   MONTREAL   SYDNEY   TOKYO

ACADEMIC PRESS INC. (LONDON) LTD.
24/28 Oval Road,
London NW1 7DX

United States Edition published by
ACADEMIC PRESS INC.
Orlando, Florida 32887

British Library Cataloguing in Publication Data
European Neuroendocrine Association (Conference :
1984 : Basle)
Dopamine and neuroendocrine active substances :
proceedings of the first symposium of the
European Neuroendocrine Association (E.N.E.A.)
Basle, Switzerland, March 4-7, 1984.
1. Endocrine glands——Diseases   2. Nervous
system——Diseases   3. Neuroendocrinology
I. Title   II. Del Pozo, Emilio   III. Flückiger,
Edward
616.8   RC648.A1

ISBN 0 12 209045 4

Printed in Great Britain

Contributors

L. F. Agnati *Department of Histology and Hormone Laboratory, Karolinska Institutet, Stockholm, Sweden.*
J. Alba-Lopez *Experimental Therapeutics Department, Sandoz Limited, Basle, Switzerland.*
J. Anderson *University of Virginia School of Medicine, Charlottesville, Virginia 22908, USA.*
K. Andersson *Department of Histology and Hormone Laboratory, Karolinska Institutet, Stockholm, Sweden.*
B. Bernardi *Department of Histology and Hormone Laboratory, Karolinska Institutet, Stockholm, Sweden.*
R. M. Blizzard *University of Virginia, Charlottesville, Virginia 22908, USA.*
D. B. Calne *Division of Neurology, University of British Columbia, Vancouver BC, Canada.*
T. Caraceni *Department of Neurology, Istituto Neurologico 'C Besta', Via Celoria 11, 20133 Milan, Italy.*
F. Cavagnini *First Medical Clinic, University of Milan, 20122 Milan, Italy.*
S. Cella *Department of Pharmacology, University of Milan, 20129 Milan, Italy.*
S. E. Christensen *Second University Clinic of Internal Medicine, Aarhus Kommunehospital, DK-8000 Aarhus C, Denmark.*
D. Cocchi *Department of Pharmacology, University of Milan, 20129 Milan, Italy.*
M. Cronin *University of Virginia School of Medicine, Charlottesville, Virginia 22908, USA.*
C. Dieguez *Department of Medicine, Welsh National School of Medicine, Heath Park, Cardiff CF4 4XN, UK.*
J. Djiane *Laboratoire de Physiologie de la Lactation, I.N.R.A., 78350 Jouy-en-Josas, France.*
P. Donatsch *Preclinical Research Department, Sandoz Limited, CH-4002 Basle, Switzerland.*
E. Dupont *University Department of Neurology, Aarhus Kommunehospital, DK-8000 Aarhus C, Denmark.*
P. Eneroth *Department of Histology and Hormone Laboratory, Karolinska Institutet, Stockholm, Sweden.*
W. S. Evans *University of Virginia, Charlottesville, Virginia 22908, USA.*
P. Falaschi *Medical Clinic V, University of Rome, 00100 Rome, Italy.*
B. de Fine Olivarius *University Department of Neurology, Aarhus Kommunehospital, DK-8000 Aarhus C, Denmark.*
S. M. Foord *Department of Medicine, Welsh National School of Medicine, Heath Park, Cardiff CF4 4XN, UK.*
L. A. Frohman *University of Cincinnati, Cincinatti, OH 45267, USA.*

R. Furlanetto *The Children's Hospital of Philadelphia, PA 19104, USA.*

K. Fuxe *Department of Histology and Hormone Laboratory, Karolinska Institutet, Stockholm, Sweden.*

P. Giovannini *Department of Neurology, Istituto Neurologico 'C Besta', Via Celoria 11, 20133 Milan, Italy.*

M. Goldstein *Department of Histology and Hormone Laboratory, Karolinska Institutet, Stockholm, Sweden.*

A. Gómez-Pan *Endocrinology Department, CNEQ Pabellon 8, Faculty of Medicine, 28040 Madrid, Spain.*

A. Guitelman *Department of Endocrinology, Hospital Alvares, Buenos Aires, Argentina.*

J. A. Gustafsson *Department of Histology and Hormone Laboratory, Karolinska Institutet, Stockholm, Sweden.*

R. Hall *Department of Medicine, Welsh National School of Medicine, Heath Park, Cardiff CF4 4XN, UK.*

A. Harfstrand *Department of Histology and Hormone Laboratory, Karolinska Institutet, Stockholm, Sweden.*

P. E. Harris *Department of Medicine, Welsh National School of Medicine, Heath Park, Cardiff CF4 4XN, UK.*

E. Hewlett *University of Virginia School of Medicine, Charlottesville, Virginia 22908, USA.*

C. Invitti *First Medical Clinic, University of Milan, 20122 Milan, Italy.*

P. B. Jorgensen *University Department of Neurology, Aarhus Kommunehospital, DK-8000 Aarhus C, Denmark.*

D. L. Kaiser *University of Virginia, Charlottesville, VA 22908, USA.*

M. Katoh *Laboratory of Molecular Endocrinology, Royal Victoria Hospital, Montreal, Quebec H3A 1A1, Canada.*

P. A. Kelly *Laboratory of Molecular Endocrinology, Royal Victoria Hospital, Montreal, Quebec H3A 1A1, Canada.*

D. Koritnik *Bowman Gray School of Medicine, Winston-Salem, North Carolina 27103, USA.*

A. Laihinen *Department of Neurology, University of Turku, SF-20520 Turku 52, Finland.*

S. W. J. Lamberts *Department of Medicine, Erasmus University, Rotterdam, The Netherlands.*

R. Landgraf, *Medizinische Klinik Innenstadt, University of Munich, 8000 Munich 2, FRG.*

P. A. LeWitt *Department of Neurology, Lafayette Clinic, 951 E Lafayette, Detroit, MI 48207, USA.*

G. Leyendecker *Department of Obstetrics and Gynecology, University of Bonn, 53 Bonn-Venusberg, FRG.*

V. Locatelli *Department of Pharmacology, University of Milan, 20129 Milan, Italy.*

P. J. Lowry *Protein Hormone Unit, St Bartholomew's Centre for Clinical Research, London EC1A 7BE, UK.*

L. Martini *Department of Endocriniology, University of Milan, 20129 Milan, Italy.*

J. H. Mendelson *Alcohol and Drug Abuse Research Center, Harvard Medical School-McLean Hospital, 115 Mill Street, Belmont, MA 02178, USA.*

N. K. Mello *Alcohol and Drug Abuse Research Center, Harvard Medical School-McLean Hospital, 115 Mill Street, Belmont, MA 02178, USA.*

D. Müller *Experimetal Therapeutics Department, Sandoz Limited, Basle, Switzerland.*

E. E. Müller *Department of Pharmacology, University of Milan, 20129 Milan, Italy.*

O. A. Müller *Medizinische Klinik Innenstadt, University of Munich, 8000 Munich 2, FRG.*

A. Neil *Department of Pharmacology, Uppsala University, Biomedical Center, Box 573, S-751 23 Uppsala, Sweden.*

R. P. Newman, *Dent Neurologic Institute, Buffalo, NR, USA.*

F. Nyberg *Department of Pharmacology, Uppsala University, Biomedical Center, Box 573, S-751 23 Uppsala, Sweden.*

R. Oeckler *Neurochirurgische Klinik Grosshadern, Frauenklinik, University of Munich, 8000 Munich 2, FRG.*

H. Orskov *Institute of Experimental Clinical Research, Aarhus Kommunehospital, DK-8000 Aarhus C, Denmark.*

E. Parati *Department of Neurology, Istituto Neurologico, 'C Besta', Via Celoria 11, 20133 Milan, Italy.*

J. R. Peters *Department of Medicine, Welsh National School of Medicine, Heath Park, Cardiff CF4 4XN, UK.*

E. Polak *Department of Endocrinology, Hospital Alvares, Buenos Aires, Argentina.*

E. Del Pozo *Experimental Therapeutics Department, Sandoz Limited, CH-4002 Basle, Switzerland.*

B. P. Richardson *Preclinical Research Department, Sandoz Limited, CH-4002 Basle, Switzerland.*

U. K. Rinne *Department of Neurology, University of Turku, SF-20520 Turku 52, Finland.*

J. Rivier *Peptide Biology Laboratory, The Salk Institute, San Diego, CA 92138-9216, USA.*

H. K. Rjosk *Frauenklinik, University of Munich, 8000 Munich 2, FRG.*

A. Rocco *Medical Clinic V, University of Rome, 00100 Rome, Italy.*

M. D. Rodriguez-Arnao, *Endocrinology Service, Hospital Provinical, 28009 Madrid, Spain.*

A. D. Rogol *University of Virginia, Charlottesville, VA 22908, USA.*

M. Rosa *Medical Clinic V, University of Rome, 00100 Rome, Italy.*

M. F. Scanlon *Department of Medicine, Welsh National School of Medicine, Heath Park, Cardiff CF4 4XN, UK.*

J. Schopohl *Medizinische Klinik Innenstadt, University of Munich, 8000 Munich 2, FRG.*

G. Scigliano *Department of Neurology, Istituto Neurologico, 'C Besta', Via Celoria 11, 20133 Milan, Italy.*

G. K. Stalla *Medizinische Klinik Innenstadt, University of Munich, 8000 Munich 2, FRG.*

L. Terenius *Department of Pharmacology, Uppsala University, Biomedical Center, Box 573, S-751 23 Uppsala, Sweden.*

M. O. Thorner *University of Virginia, Charlottesville, VA 22908, USA.*

G. Tolis *Division of Endocrinology, Hippokrateion Hospital, 115 27 Athens, Greece.*

W. Vale *Peptide Biology Laboratory, The Salk Institute, San Diego, CA 92138-9216, USA.*

W. Vale   *Department of Histology and Hormone Laboratory, Karolinska Institutet, Stockholm, Sweden.*

M. L. Vance   *University of Virginia, Charlottesville, VA 22908, USA.*

K. Von Werder   *Medizinische Klinik Innenstadt, University of Munich, 8000 Munich 2, FRG.*

L. Wildt   *Department of Obstetrics and Gynecology, University of Bonn, 53 Bonn-Venusberg, FRG.*

M. Wills   *Department of Medicine, University of Virginia School of Medicine, Charlottesville, Virginia, USA.*

Z. Y. Yu   *Department of Histology and Hormone Laboratory, Karolinska Institutet, Stockholm, Sweden.*

A. Yotis   *Division of Endocrinology, Hippokrateion Hospital, 115 27 Athens, Greece.*

Contents

Part I
Dopamine and Pituitary Hormones

Part II
Neuroendocrine Aspects of Neurological Disease

Part III
Prolactin and Dopamine Agonists

Part IV
Control of Gonadotropin Release

Part V
Opiates: Neuroendocrine Correlations and Pain

Part VI
Advances in Brain Peptide Research

PREFACE

This volume comprises the invited reports delivered at the 1st Meeting of the European Neuroendocrine Association (E.N.E.A.) in Basel (4-7, March 1984). The reports present neuroendocrine advances both in laboratory work and at the clinical level, and they cover a wide spectrum of physiological, pathophysiological and pharmacological interests. This encompasses neurohistological aspects of the hypothalamo-pituitary axis, neuromodulators, neurotransmitters, as well as aspects of receptors on hormonal target cells. Rapid progress in separate fields have contributed to the present day understanding of neuroendocrine mechanisms, from the molecular level to the organismic level. It was therefore felt necessary to bring together these different but interrelated areas of work under the common denominator of the European Neuroendocrine Association. It was hoped that such a meeting would facilitate a stimulating exchange of knowledge and speculations. During the E.N.E.A. Meeting the positive aspects of such an interdisciplinary approach as this conference provided were felt very strongly by many participants. In reading the chapters of this volume this impression is revived.

A collection of further reports with a heavier bias towards neurological aspects and problems will be published in a separate volume.

E. del Pozo   E. Flückiger

I. Dopamine and Pituitary Hormones

PHARMACOLOGY OF DOPAMINOMIMETIC DRUGS

E. Flückiger

Pharmaceutical Division, Preclinical Research
SANDOZ LTD.,
CH-4002 Basel, Switzerland

INTRODUCTION

It seems of interest to note that dopamine pharmacology developed in two distinct phases. In the fifties and sixties it was the aspect of dopamine antagonism (neuroleptics) and now in the seventies and eighties it is dopamine receptor agonists which attract so much attention. Both phases were successfully opened by phenomenological pharmacology, receptor pharmacology being a more recent chapter.

Although it was recognized already in the fifties that neuroleptics (dopamine antagonists) have endocrine effects (e.g. galactorrhea in patients treated with chlorpromazine (43), experimental induction of lactation in rabbits with the same drug (2), this had little consequences in pharmacological endocrinology, with the notable exception of Sulman's attempt to select prolactin stimulating drugs lacking central sedative effects (for review: see 40). Shelesnyak in an entirely different context but simultaneously discovered and explored the prolactin secretion inhibitory property of ergot alkaloids (e.g. 38; 39; 26), again with no immediate echo in pharmacological endocrinology. The scene became activated at the beginning of the seventies when bromocriptine, which had been selected and developed for clinical use as a prolactin secretion inhibitor pure and simple (15; 12) was demonstrated in the rat to have central dopamine agonist activity (20; 24; 8), to be of benefit in M. Parkinson patients (4, 5) and to lower circulating growth hormone levels in acromegalic patients (28). Both these effects were explained to be related to its direct dopaminomimetic property, and a few years later it became certain that prolactin secretion inhibition also was due to this property (29). In the past ten years the pharmacology of do-

paminomimetics has developed in various directions, the major
ones being: receptor characterization (by biochemical, bio-
physical, physico-chemical, anatomical, behavioural criteria),
target cell physiology, drug chemistry.

DOPAMINE RECEPTORS

Experimental evidence indicates that dopamine receptors
function in many regulatory systems and that they occur in
various subtypes, differing not only by anatomic criteria
(autoreceptors, pre- and postsynaptic receptors) but also by
biochemical and functional criteria (such as being linked to
an adenylate cyclase system in a inhibitory or excitatory way,
or not being linked to adenylate cyclase) or by physico-chemical criteria (radioligand studies). Dopamine receptor typing
is *in statu nascendi*, and quite naturally this makes it difficult to the mere observer of the scene to gain a clear overview. For the case of the dopamine receptors in the CNS this
is greatly helped by a recent review (27). For an overview on
peripheral dopamine receptors, mainly considering the vascular
system, there also exists a recent review (21). It is apparent
from the literature that important differences still exist
between the various views on dopamine receptors subtypes.

Of endocrine cells equipped with dopamine receptors only
three cell types have been analyzed in detail, the prolactin
producing cells of the anterior pituitary lobe, the MSH producing cells of the intermediate pituitary lobe and the PTH
producing cells of the parathyroid gland. Comparing the pharmacology of the prolactin and the PTH cell led to the proposition by Kebabian and Calne (25) of D_1 and D_2 dopamine receptor which transduces a stimulatory signal to an adenylate
cyclase system with the PTH cell as the prototype. The D_2 receptor being a dopamine receptor which is not linked to adenylate cyclase, with the prolactin cell as the prototype. Further experience though demonstrated that dopaminergic stimulation of both the prolactin and the MSH producing cell leads
to a reduction of cAMP content trough inhibition of the adenylate cyclase system (33; 9; 34). The D_1 receptor thus transduces a stimulatory, the D_2 receptor an inhibitory dopaminergic
signal.

Dopamine receptors on other dopamine responsive endocrine
cells such as the TSH producing cells of the rat anterior pituitary, the ACTH producing human pituitary adenoma cells or
the aldosterone producing rat adrenal glomerulosa cells still
are only superficially characterized (13). Evidence exists
that dopamine receptors in human pituitary adenoma cells may
be heterogenous (13) as evidenced by unexpected results from

radioligand studies (3).

DRUGS

In recent years more than 20 different research groups have published new dopaminomimetic compounds. Many of these compounds, including the classical ergot compounds or ergoline derivatives contain in their structure the phenylethylamine moiety of dopamine (14). This moiety is considered by many as essential for dopaminomimetic activity. But this view is too narrow as demonstrated by the existence of such recognized dopaminomimetics as piribedil, a piperazine, as EMD 23 448, an indolyl-3-butylamide (37).

Structure activity relationship (SAR) studies have been performed in various structural groups and their results have recently been admirably discussed (6). The review concludes that SAR of dopamine agonists are "exquisitely subtle and are not yet understood". Goals of synthetic work by the various research groups have been several: to increase potency and or duration of action, to create selective dopaminomimetics (if possible for one subtype of dopamine receptors), to find new patentable structures. Progress toward the three goals has certainly been achieved (see e.g. Table 1), but very few compounds have reached the stage of clinical application.

TABLE 1

Subtype-selective dopamine receptor agonists

Compound, Code name	Chemistry	Specificity	Reference
1) SKF 38393	tetrahydrobenzazepines	D_1 receptor	35
2) Ly 141865	reduced ergoline structure: pyrazoloquinoline	D_2 receptor	41
3) 3-PPP	phenylpiperidines	autoreceptor	23
4) TL-99	aminotetralines	autoreceptor	22
5) RDS-127	indeamines	autoreceptor	1

We have understandably spent much time to study the pharmacological profile of modifications on the bromocriptine
molecule. As an example Figure 1 presents the subcutaneous
activity of such compounds on the rat ovum implantation inhibition test in percent of the activity of bromocriptine.
Only single chemical changes are considered here. Figure 1
shows that not only changes in various positions of the ergoline structure (numbered 1-14) but also changes at the
"periphery", in the cyclopeptide moiety (positions numbered
1'-11') influence biological potency in an important way. Very
few changes were favorable to the *in vivo* potency. Figure 2
demonstrates detailed pharmacological activities of a number
of homologues in position 6 of bromocriptine (18). It is interesting to note that increasing F from methyl to ethyl
changed the antagonist property of bromocriptine at the D_1
receptor to agonist activity. This new property together with
an increased potency in the implantation inhibition test, was
accompanied by no change in affinity to striatal ^{3}H-dopamine
and ^{3}-spiroperidol binding sites, no increased emetic potency

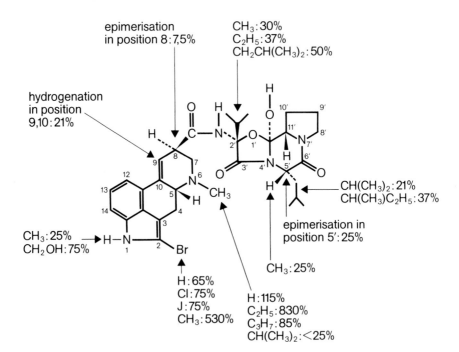

*Fig. 1. Bromocriptine derivatives I: Effects of single chem-
ical changes to the bromocriptine molecule on relative prolactin inhibitory activity in vivo.*

but reduced motor effects. These qualitative changes in the profile of actions were unexpected and they are of great interest for reflections on SAR.

Similar work was done with amino-ergolines, starting from compound CH 29-717, N,N-dimethyl-N'-(6-methyl-ergoline-8α-yl)-sulfamide hydrochloride (16). In Figure 3 the structure of this compound is indicated together with the prolactin secretion inhibitory potency (as assessed *in vivo* in the classical implantation inhibition test) of CH 29-717 and some of its derivatives. In Table 2 the dopaminomimetic profiles of selected compounds of this series as assessed *in vivo* and *in vitro* are compared.

Of these CU 32-085 is of special interest (17; 19). The serum prolactin lowering potency of CU 32-085 was 40 times lower at 1 hour after s.c. administration than that of CH 29-717. At 2 hours CU 32-085 was 14 times weaker and at 8 and 24 hours 2 times less potent than CH 29-717. In the brain of treated rats DOPAC concentration was first increased after CU 32-085, indicating acceleration of DA turnover, and the

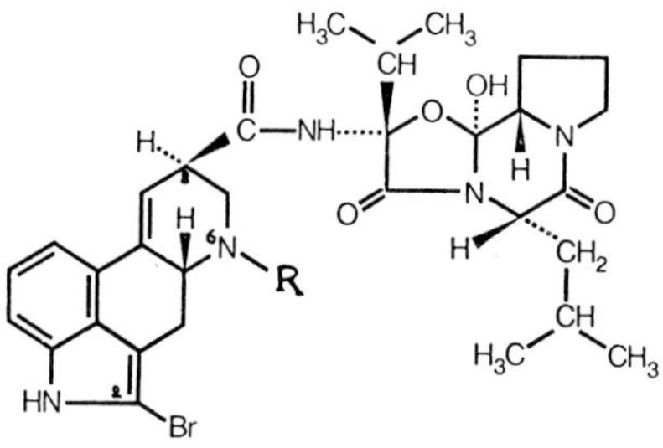

Effects	R= -H	-CH$_3$	-CH$_2$ CH$_3$	-CH$_2$ CH$_2$CH$_3$	-CH (CH$_3$)$_2$	-CH$_2$ CH$_2$CH$_2$CH$_3$	-CH$_2$ CH$_2$CH$_2$CH$_2$CH$_3$
Implant.inhib.rat, ED$_{50}$ mg/kg s.c.	0.65	0.75	0.09	0.88	>3	>3	>3
Ungerstedt rat, MED, mg/kg s.c.	>10	0.1	>10	>3	>1	>1	>1
Stereotyped behav. rat, MED, mg/kg i.p.	30	0.5	30	>30	30	30	30
DA sens.aden.cyclase +agonist, -antagonist	-	+			+	(-)	(-)
Striatal affinity (binding) IC$_{50}$ (nM) DA/SP		48/13	73/13		650/24		
Emesis, dog, ED$_{50}$ µg/kg i.v.		7.5	5.8				
5-HT sens.aden.cyclase +agonist, -antagonist	-	+			+	(-)	(-)
A.basilaris (5-HT) +agonist, -antagonist	->+	-+					

Fig. 2. Bromocriptine derivatives II: Effect of homologuous changes at position 6 of the molecule on the profile of activities.

expected decrease became evident only after 4 hours. This
biphasic effect indicates that CU 32-085 in the brain first
acted as an antagonist and only later as an agonist (10).
This could be confirmed by detailed *ex vivo* biochemical
studies in the rat (12). Further it was found that *in
vitro* CU 32-085 is an antagonist at D_1 (μM range), and
also an antagonist at D_2 receptors in the nM range (32).
CU 32-085 added to primary pituitary cell cultures produced only a slight inhibition of prolactin release (D_2
agonistic action at 10^{-7} and 10^{-6}M, but when incubated
together with CH 29-717 antagonized dose dependently the
activity of the latter (30).

CU 32-085 therefore is mainly a dopamine antagonist which
is metabolically converted to a full dopamine agonist. One
urinary metabolite, 1,20-N,N-bisdemethylated, was found to
slow brain dopamine metabolism monophasically (11) and to
stimulate both D_1 and D_2 receptors at micromolar and nano-
molar concentrations, respectively (32).

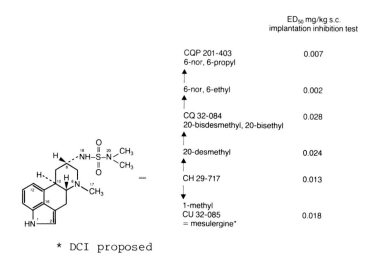

* DCI proposed

*Fig. 3. 8α-amino-ergolines. Structural changes and changes
in activity to suppress prolactin secretion in vivo. For
further activities see Table 2.*

TABLE 2

Comparison of dopaminomimetic potencies

Test	CB 154	CH 29-717	CQ 32-084	CU 32-085
1) Inhibition of radio- ligand binding calf caudate IC_{50} (nM) ^{3}H-DA/^{3}H-spiro	84/13	210/120	120/25	1400/140
2) Prl↓, ♂ rat (2hr) ID_{50} (µg/kg s.c.)	8	0.9	5	10
3) Ungerstedt rat MED (µg/kg s.c.)	100	50	10	300
4) HF↓ cat ID_{50} (µg/kg i.v.)	15	3.4	5.8	45
5) DA-AC rat striatum E/pD$_2$ PK$_i$	∅ 6.4	∅ <5	32/5.8 ∅	∅ 6.3
6) Ach release↓ rat striatum	5	5	2.5	1580
7) DA release↓ rat striatum	ag/(nM)	?	ag(µM)	antag

References to methods used: Test 1: Closse *et al.* (1980) (7) who kindly contributed these results. Test 2: Flückiger *et al.* (1979) (17). Test 3: Vigouret *et al.* (1978) (42). Test 4: Scholtysik and Müller-Schweinitzer (1980) (36). Test 5-7: Markstein (1981) (31).

MED = minimal effective dose; HF = heart frequency; DA-AC = dopamine sensitive adenylate cyclase; Ach = acetylcholine; E_r = relative efficacy in % of maximal DA effect; pD_2 = log EC_{50}; pK_i = log K_{diss}.

REFERENCES

1. Arneric, J.P., Long, J.P., Williams, M., Goodale, D.B., Lakoski, G.M. and Gebhart, G.F. (1983). *J. Pharmacol. Exp. Ther.* **224**, 161-169.
2. Audibert, A., Forgue, G. and Gage, C.(1956). *C.R.Soc.Biol.* (Paris) **150**, 173-175.
3. Bression, D., Brandi, A.M., Nousbaum, A., LeDafniet, M., Racadot, J. and Peillon , F. (1982). *J. Clin. Endocrinol. Metab.* **55**, 589-593.
4. Calne, D.B., Teychenne, P.F., Claveria, L.E., Eastman, R., Greenacre, J.K. and Petrie, A. (1974a). *Br. Med. J.* **4**, 442-444.
5. Calne, D.B., Teychenne, P.F., Leigh, P.N., Banji, A.N. and Greenacre, J.K. (1974b). *Lancet* **2**, 1355-1356.
6. Cannon, J.G. (1983). *Ann. Rev. Pharmacol. Toxicol.* **23**, 103-130.
7. Closse, A., Frick, W., Hauser, D. and Sauter, A. (1980). *In* "Psychopharmacology and Biochemistry of Neurotransmitter Receptors (Eds H.I. Yamamura, R.W. Olsen and E. Usdin), pp. 463-474. Elsevier/North Holland, Amsterdam.
8. Corrodi, H., Fuxe, K., Hökfelt, T., Lidbrink, P. and Ungerstedt, U. (1973). *J. Pharm. Pharmacol.* **25**, 409-411.
9. Cronin, M.J. and Thorner, M.O. (1982). *J. Cyclic Nucleotide Res.* **8**, 267-275.
10. Enz, A. (1981) *Life Sci.* **29**, 2227-2234.
11. Enz, A., Frick, W., Closse, A., Nordmann, R. and Palacios, J.M. (1982). "Abstracts", 13th CINP Congress, Jerusalem, **1**, 199.
12. Flückiger, E. (1972). *In* "Prolactin and Carcinogenesis" (Eds A.R. Boyns and K. Griffiths), pp. 162-171. Alpha Omega Alpha Publishing, Cardiff (UK).
13. Flückiger, E. (1983). *J. Neural Transm.* suppl. **18**, 189-205.
14. Flückiger, E. (1984). "3rd European Workshop on Pituitary Adenomas, Amsterdam 1983" (Eds S.W.J. Lamberts *et al.)* (in press).
15. Flückiger, E. and Wagner, H.-R. (1968). *Experientia* **24**, 1130-1131.
16. Flückiger, E., Briner, U., Doepfner, W., Kovacs, E., Marbach, P. and Wagner, H.-R. (1978). *Experientia* **34**, 1330-1331.
17. Flückiger, E., Briner, U., Bürki, H.R., Marbach, P., Wagner, H.-R. and Doepfner, W. (1979). *Experientia* **35**, 1677-1678.

18. Flückiger, E., Doepfner, W., Jaton, A.L., Markstein, R., Müller-Schweinitzer, E. and Wagner, H.-R. (1981). *Experientia* 37, 669.
19. Flückiger, E., Briner, U., Enz, A., Markstein, R. and Vigouret, J.M. (1983). *In* "Lisuride and Other Dopamine Agonists" (Eds D.B. Calne, R. Horowski, R.J. McDonald, W. Wuttke), pp. 1-9. Raven Press, New York.
20. Fuxe, K. and Hökfelt, T. (1970). *In* "The Hypothalamus" (Eds L. Martini, M. Motta, F. Fraschini), pp. 123-138. Academic Press, New York.
21. Goldberg, L.I. and Kohli, J.D. (1983). *In* "Dopamine Receptor Agonists 1" (Eds A. Carlsson and J.L.G. Nilsson), pp. 92-98. Pharmaceutical Press, Stockholm.
22. Goodale, D.B., Rusterholz, D.B., Long, J.P., Flynn, J.R., Walsh, B., Cannon, J.G. and Lee, T. (1980). *Science* 210, 1141-1143.
23. Hjorth, S.A., Carlsson, A., Wilkstrom, H., Lindberg, P., Sanches, D., Hacksell, U., Arvidsson, L.E., Svensson, U. and Nilsson, J.L.G. (1981). *Life Sci.* 28, 1225-1238.
24. Hökfelt, T. and Fuxe, K. (1972). *In* "Brain Endocrine Interactions: Median Eminence: Structure and Function" (Eds K.M. Knigge, D.E. Scott and A. Weindl), pp. 181-223. Karger, Basel.
25. Kebabian, J.W. and Calne, D.B. (1979). *Nature* 277, 93.
26. Kraicer, P.F. and Shelesnyak, M.C. (1965). *J. Reprod. Fertil.* 10, 221-226.
27. Leff, S.E. and Cresse, I. (1983). *TIPS* 6, 463-467.
28. Liuzzi, A., Chiodini, P.G., Botalla, L., Cremascoli, G., Müller, E.E. and Silvestrini, F. (1974). *J. Clin. Endocrinol. Metab.* 38, 910-912.
29. McLeod, R.M. (1976). *In* "Frontiers in Neuroendocrinology" (Eds L. Martini and W.F. Ganong). Vol. IV, pp. 169-194. Raven Press, New York.
30. Markó, M. (1984). *Eur. J. Pharmacol.* 101, 263-266.
31. Markstein, R. (1981). *J. Neural Transm.* 51, 39-59.
32. Markstein, R. (1983). *Eur. J. Pharmacol.* 95, 101-107.
33. Markstein, R., Herrling, P.L. and Wagner, H.R. (1978). "Proc. VIIth Internat. Congress of Pharmacology" (IUPHAR) (Paris), Abstract 23-26. Pergamon Press, Oxford.
34. Munemura, M., Cote, T.E., Tsuruta, K., Eskay, R.L. and Kebabian, J.W. (1980). *Endocrinology* 107, 1676-1683.
35. Setler, P.E., Saran, H.M., Zirkle, C.L. and Saunders, H.L. (1978). *Eur. J. Pharmacol.* 50, 419-430.
36. Scholtysik, G. and Müller-Schweinitzer, E. (1980). *In* "Modulation of Neurochemical Transmission" (Ed. E.S.

THE EXTERNAL LAYER OF THE MEDIAN EMINENCE AND THE PARAVENTRIC-
ULAR HYPOTHALAMIC NUCLEUS REPRESENT TWO IMPORTANT LEVELS OF
INTEGRATION IN THE NEUROENDOCRINE REGULATION. STUDIES ON PEP-
TIDE-CATECHOLAMINE INTERACTIONS GIVE EVIDENCE FOR THE
EXISTENCE OF "MEDIANOSOMES"

K. Fuxe, L.F. Agnati, K. Andersson, P. Eneroth, A. Härfstrand, M. Goldstein, B. Bernardi, W. Vale, Z.-Y. Yu and
J.-A. Gustafsson

*Department of Histology and Hormone Laboratory,
Karolinska Institutet, Stockholm, Sweden*

INTRODUCTION

Based on studies using quantitative chemical neuro-
anatomy we have during recent years introduced the hypothesis that the local circuits in the external layer of the
median eminence represent one important intergrative ele-
ment in the regulation of the release of hypothalamic hormones from the median eminence (1). Noradrenaline (NA)
and especially dopamine (DA) nerve terminals represent
important elements in the local circuits of the external
layer of the median eminence. In addition, DA is released
as a prolactin inhibitor factor (PIF) from the medial pa-
lisade zone (MPZ) of the median eminence. The hormonal
properties of DA in the MPZ may explain the presence of
a D_1 DA receptor in the median eminence, which is of a
low affinity type. In fact, a high affinity type of DA
receptor should be constantly saturated in view of the
high local concentration of the hormonally released DA
from the MPZ (2). In the present paper we will further
define the role of DA and NA in the intergrative functions of the local circuits of the median eminence.

Another important level of integration in the regulation of the release of hypothalamic hormones is the soma-
dendritic level of the peptidergic neurons, especially
within the nucleus paraventricularis hypothalami (PA)

DOPAMINE AND NEUROENDOCRINE
ACTIVE SUBSTANCES
ISBN 0 12 209045 4

(3,4). In this paper we will analyze the morphological
interactions between NA and A nerve terminals, CRF neurons
and glucocorticoid receptors in this nucleus.

RESULTS

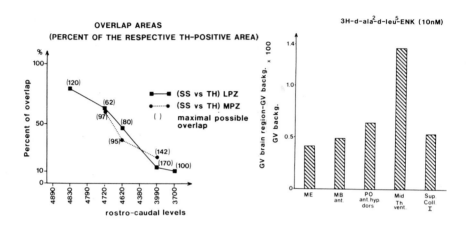

*Fig. 1. Overlap areas between SS and TH immunoreactive areas
in the MPZ and LPZ. The figures in parenthesis indicate the
theoretical maximal overlap which is possible.*
*Fig. 3. Measurement of gray values by means of image analysis
of receptor autoradiograms using the delta-opiate receptor
radioligand.*

Morphological and Morphometrical Studies

Median eminence level: Based on morphometrical studies
it has been concluded that the DA and LHRH nerve terminals
in the LPZ may be organized in mediolateral "domains" or
"medianosomes" extending in the entire rostrocaudal direction, being involved with the release of one type of hypothalamic hormone and having a differential regulation (5).
However, studies on the morphological interaction (overlap
areas) between somatostatin (SRIF) and DA nerve terminals
in the LPZ and MPZ at various rostrocaudal levels of the
median eminence (fig. 1.) indicate that these medianosomes
mainly operate at rostral levels in the MPZ and LPZ, indicating the existence also of a rostrocaudal subdivision.
Large numbers of SRIF terminals are not regulated by DA
terminals.
Paraventricular hypothalamic level: The close morphological interaction and the large overlap between A (PNMT)
immunoreactive networks, the glucocorticoid receptor (GR)

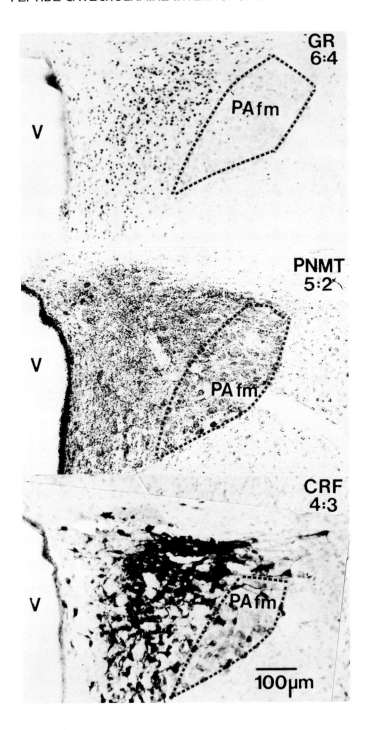

Fig. 2. Glucocorticoid receptor PNMT and CRF immunoreactivity is shown in adjacent vibrotome sections of the nucleus paraventricularis hypothalami.

immunoreactive and the CRF immunoreactive nerve cell bodies
of the parvocellular part is shown (Fig. 2). It seems likely
that many of the CRF immunoreactive neurons contain glucocorticoid receptors (see 6). Thus, neurons can be regulated
not only by high densities of A nerve terminals and by their
contents of GR (see Fig. 2).

QUANTITATIVE RECEPTOR STUDIES

By the use of the DA receptor radioligand ^{3}H-flupenthixol
and ^{3}H-fluphenazine and computer assisted microdensitometry
the existence of a DA receptor of the D_1 type in the rat
median eminence has been indicated, since these radioligands
strongly label the median eminence in the presence of D-2 and
α_1 receptor antagonists (see also 2). The existence of opiate
receptors in the median eminence has been shown by use of
the ^{3}H-etorphine radioligand which labels the μtype of opiate
receptor, and the radioligand ^{3}H-d-ala[2]-H-d-leu[5]-enkephaline
(DALE), which labels the delta type of opiate receptor. Both
[3]H-etorphine (1 and 4 nm) and ^{3}H-DALE (4 nM) weakly but significantly labels the entire median eminence in its rostrocaudal extent. However, the μ receptor is especially present
in the caudal half (Fig. 3). Hence, μ and delta type of opiate
receptors may operate although in low densities together with
the high densities of D_1 receptors in the local circuits of
the median eminence.

The D-1 receptor agonist, SKF 38-393 has failed to modulate
DA levels and DA turnover within the median eminence probably
due to the failure of the D-1 agonist to induce a transneuronal
feedback as well as to the relative absence of DA autoreceptors.
As seen the D-1 agonist produced a significant increase of
prolactin secretion, while the LH secretion was not significantly affected. These results indicate the possibility that
the D-1 receptor may inhibit the secretion of another PIF such
as GABA. Furthermore, SKF 38-393 following systemic treatment
may, due to its pharmacokinetic properties, exert mixed DA
agonistic and antagonistic actions on D-1 receptors. Such a
property may explain its failure to consistently modulate LH
secretion in the male rat.

QUANTITATIVE MICROFLUORIMETRICAL STUDIES

Effect of hypothalamic factors on CA levels. LHRH in a dose
of 100μg/kg selectively increases DA turnover in the LPZ
of the median eminence and reduces NA turnover in the
nucleus preopticus medialis (POM) (see 4,7). TRH in a dose

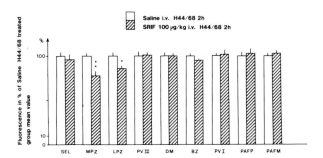

Fig. 4.

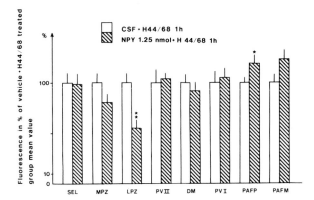

Fig. 5.

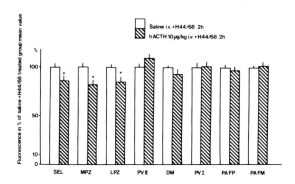

Fig. 6.

Figs. 4 - 6. Disappearance of CA fluorescene following i.v. SRIF (Fig. 4) and hACTH (Fig. 6) injection in the hypophysectomized male rat and an i.v.t. injection of NPY into the normal male rat (Fig. 5) immediately following TH inhibition using α-methyl tyrosine methyl ester (H44/68, 250 mg/* = p <0.05; ** = p <0.01.)

of 10 - 100 μg/kg increases the DA turnover in the MPZ and
LPZ and reduces NA turnover in both the PA fp and PA fm
(5). CRF increases NA turnover in the subependymal layer
(SEL) and in the MPZ and reduces NA turnover in the PA
fp, PA fm and the anterior periventricular area (PV I).
SRIF (100 μg/kg) increases DA turnover both in the MPZ and
LPZ (Fig. 4). These results have led us to believe that
there exist in the respective "medianosomes" of the
median eminence reciprocal synapses between LHRH and DA
boutons, between TRH and DA boutons, between CRF and NA
boutons, and between SRIF and DA boutons (4). It is
possible that the ultrashort feedback action of
hypothalamic hormones may involve a neuronal mechanism,
which at least in part consists of reciprocal synapses,
through which a prompt reduction of hypothalamic hormone
release may be produced via the increased release of DA or
NA. However, it must be considered that e.g. SRIF
terminals also surround DA cell bodies in the arcuate
nucleus. Therefore, this level of regulation of DA neurons
by SRIF and other hypothalamic hormones can also be of
importance. In view of the blood-brain barrier it is
postulated that the changes in the NA turnover observed in
discrete parts of the hypothalamus, especially within PA
after systemic injection of hypothalamic hormones, are
caused by the existence of neuronal feedback loops from
the medial basal hypothalamus into e.g. POM and PA
respectively. These loops are activated by receptors for
hypothalamic hormones belonging to recurrent collaterals
of the respective hypothalamic hormone containing systems
innnervating the median eminence. In this way information
of activity in the medial basal hypothalamus and within
the median eminence may reach back into the somatodendritic area of the peptidergic neurons, which is controlled
by local circuits in which especially NA and A nerve terminals participate. The results are in agreement with the
view that NA nerve terminals exert an excitatory influence
on LHRH, TRH and CRF neuronal activity in view of the
demonstration of reduced NA turnovers in POM and PA respectively, following the i.v. injection of LHRH (POM), TRH
(PA) and CRF (PA).

Effects of other neuropeptides: Another neuropeptide,
neuropeptide Y (NPY) has been discovered to selectively
and markedly increase DA turnover in LPZ and to reduce NA
turnover in PA (Fig. 5). NPY immunoreactive nerve cell
bodies and nerve terminal networks in high densities have
been demonstrated within the arcuate nucleus (see 8) indicating that NPY immunoreactive terminals may directly

regulate the tuberoinfundibular DA neurons at the level of
the arcuate nucleus (9). High densities of NPY terminals
are found in the PA, where NPY may be a comodulator in CA
terminals. NPY reduced significantly the secretion of
prolactin and LH and produced a marked increase in the
secretion of corticosterone. These endocrine effects were
abolished by the presence of tyrosine hydroxylase inhibition and may in part be mediated via increased DA release
(prolactin, LH). In agreement with the present findings
another pancreatripolypeptide PYY has been found to produce similar effects on both CA turnover and on the secretion of anterior pituitary hormones (9). These results
further amplify the large numbers of discrete peptide
monoamine interactions which appear to exist in the inte-
grative processes controlling the release of hypothalamic
hormones.

*Effects of rat prolactin, rat GH, rat TSH, ACTH 1 - 24
and human ACTH on CA turnover in the hypophysectomized
male rat.* (See 1,4). Each anterior pituitary hormone in-
duces its own pattern of turnover changes of CA in the
median eminence. Thus, rat prolactin acutely (100 μg/kg,
i.v.) selectively increases DA turnover in the MPZ, while
rat TSH (10 - 100 μg/kg, i.v.) increase DA turnover in
both the MPZ and LPZ of the median eminence. Rat GH (100
μg/kg, i.v.) instead reduces DA turnover in the MPZ and
LPZ and reduces NA turnover in the SEL, while ACTH 1-24
selectively increases NA turnover in the SEL and MPZ and
ACTH increases both NA (MPZ, SEL) and DA turnover (LPZ) in
the median eminence (Fig. 6). Thus, ACTH may when released
in stress turn off the secretion of LH and TSH via increasing DA release e.g. by interfering with the action of the
ACTH-β-endorphin system in its regulation of the tuberoinfundibular DA neurons to the LPZ. All these studies
suggest that the short feedback action of pituitary hormones may in part be mediated via membrane receptors present
in the local circuits of the respective "medianosomes" of
the median eminence and which may modulate peptide release
at least to a major extent via regulation of DA and/or NA
synthesis and release in the respective "medianosomes".

   However, all the pituitary hormones also induced highly
discrete changes of NA levels and/or turnover in discrete
hypothalamic regions containing the hypothalamic hormone
containing cell bodies. In view of the brain barrier these
actions may be mediated as indicated above via neuronal
feedback loops into the somatodendritic regions of hypothalamic hormone producing pathways. These neural feedback
loops may in a highly discrete way be regulated by recep-

tors for pituitary hormones within the mediobasal hypothalamus and partly exert this feedback action by modulation
of NA release in the local circuits respective area. The
NA terminals in PA may also coordinate responses within
the various peptidergic populations of the paraventricular
hypothalamic nucleus in order to obtain a proper pattern
of changes of release of pituitary hormones both from the
anterior and posterior pituitary gland.

REFERENCES

1. Andersson, K., Fuxe, K., Eneroth, P., Agnati, L.F. and
    Locatelli, V. (1980). *In* "Progress in Psychoneuroendo-
    crinology"(Eds F. Brambilla, G. Racagni and D. de
    Wied), pp. 395-406. Elsevier, Amsterdam.
2. Fuxe, K., Agnati, L.F., Benfenati, F., Andersson, K.,
    Camurri, M. and Zoli, M. (1983). *Neurosci. Lett.* <u>44</u>,
    185-190.
3. Fuxe, K., Hökfelt, T., Johansson, O., Ganten, D., Gold-
    stein, M., Perez de la Mora, M., Possani, L., Tapia,
    R., Teran, L., Palacios, R., Said, S. and Mutt, V.
    (1976). *In* "Colloque de Synthèse 1976, Série Action
    Thématique Rapport No. 7: Action Thématique 22 et 35,
    Neuroendocrinologie", pp. 17-40, INSERM, Paris.
4. Fuxe, K., Agnati, L.F., Calza, L., Andersson, K.,
    Giardino, L., Benfenati, F., Camurri, M. and Gold-
    stein, M. (1984). *In* "Neurology and Neurobiology",
    Vol. 8B (Catecholamines: Part B. Neuropharmacology and
    CNS: Theoretical Aspects)(Ed. E. Usdin). Alan R. Liss
    Inc., New York.
5. Calza, L., Agnati, L.F., Fuxe, K., Giardino, L. and
    Goldstein, M. (1983). *Neurosci. Lett.* <u>43</u>, 179-183.
6. Fuxe, K., Agnati, L.F., Härfstrand, A., Yu, Z.-Z., Okret,
    S., Wilkström, A.-C., Granholm, S., Zoli, M., Vale,
    W. and Gustafsson, J.-A. (1984). *Proc. Natl. Acad.
    Sci.* (in press).
7. Andersson, K. and Eneroth, P. (1984). *Eur. J. Pharmacol.*
    (in press).
8. Hökfelt, T., Everitt, B.J., Theodorsson-Norheim, E.,
    Terenius, L., Tatemoto, K., Mutt, Va. and Goldstein,
    M. (1984). *In* "Neurology and Neurobiology", Vol. 8B
    (Catecholamines: Part. B. Neuropharmacology and CNS:
    Theoretical Aspects)(Ed. E. Usind). Alan R. Liss Inc.,
    New York.
9. Fuxe, K., Andersson, K., Agnati, L.F., Eneroth, P.,
    Locatelli, V., Cavicchioli, L., Mascagni, F., Tate-
    moto, K. and Mutt, V. (1982). *Inserm* <u>110</u>, 65-86.

THE DOPAMINE RECEPTOR IN THE ANTERIOR PITUITARY GLAND

M. Cronin*, J. Anderson*, D. Koritnik[+] and E. Hewlett*

*University of Virginia School of Medicine
Charlottesville, Virginia 22908, USA

[+]Bowman Gray School of Medicine
Winston-Salem, North Carolina 27103, USA

INTRODUCTION

In the anterior pituitary gland (AP), more is currently known about the dopamine (DA) receptor than the other receptor types. Radioligand binding techniques have enabled extensive characterization of this entity in membranes, cytosol, whole cells and tumors derived from the AP of a variety of mammals (1, 2, 3, reviewed in 4 & 5). Unfortunately, little is documented in primate tissue to allow any degree of confidence when extrapolating subprimate data to man. We were fortunate to acquire enough monkey AP to determine if the pharmacological profile of DA receptor binding was analogous to that observed in the bovine and porcine AP.

The AP DA receptor was initially classified as the D-2 subtype, in part because investigators assumed it was not coupled to adenylate cyclase, a treacherous speculation that is no longer tenable. DA receptor activation is now known to inhibit adenylate cyclase activity and cyclic AMP (cAMP) accumulation in the AP (6, referenced in 7). With this observation established, we have applied to the AP complimentary probes that perturb specific components of the cAMP-generating system. By so doing, the sufficiency of several cell membrane proteins for the coordinated response to DA receptor activation was addressed.

The agents used include pertussis toxin (PT) protein, which is synthesized by the bacterium Bordatella pertussis. This exotoxin covalently modifies a cell membrane protein postulated to mediate hormone-receptor initiated inhibition of adenylate cyclase activity, the so-called N_i protein. The result is functional attenuation of inhibitory receptor systems linked to adenylate cyclase (reviewed in 8). Indeed, we showed that PT treatment of AP cells blocked DA inhibition of cAMP accumulation and prolactin release (7). The other probe used was forskolin, which appears to stimulate directly the catalytic subunit of adenylate cyclase (9). This diterpene amplifies cAMP accumulation in and prolactin release from AP cells (10). Thus, it was of theoretical interest to analyze the reaction of forskolin-treated cells to DA and PT.

MATERIALS AND EXPERIMENTAL METHODS

AP membranes from cyanomologous monkeys were prepared and ^{3}H-spiperone (45 Ci/mmol; New England Nuc.) binding was conducted as previously described (1). Primary cultures of male rat AP were established (11), whereas in the hemolytic plaque assay, recently dispersed cells were cultured for 2–6 days before being applied to Cunningham chambers as described elsewhere (12). The plaques were developed for 45 min at 37C with 1:50 dilutions of guinea pig complement and anti-rat prolactin (rab) serum #AFPC2381. PT was prepared (8) and added to cultured cells at 70 ng/ml for at least 24 hr, a time producing maximal effects in a variety of cell types. Butaclamol (Ayerst), bromocriptine (Sandoz), pergolide (Lilly) and somatostatin (Drs. Ling & Guillemin, California) were generous gifts. Forskolin, and other DA agents were purchased from commercial sources. Radioimmunoassays quantitated the amounts of prolactin (measured in the laboratory of Dr. R. MacLeod) and cAMP (measured in the DRTC Core Lab). The data were evaluated statistically with an analysis of variance with a Neuman-Keuls test.

RESULTS

The binding of the DA antagonist ^{3}H-spiroperidol to AP membranes from *Macaca fascicularis* monkeys is pharmacologically similar to the data obtained with other mammals (Fig. 1). This finding confers some confidence in extrapolating to primate the conclusions drawn from the majority of binding data obtained in the rat, ovine and porcine AP.

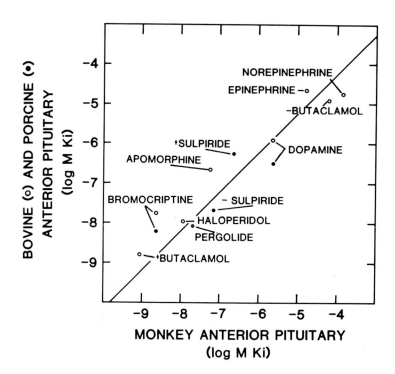

Fig. 1. Agonists and antagonists competed against ^{3}H-spiperone binding to DA receptors in particulate preparations of the AP. The concentration of various agents necessary to displace half of the binding (K_i) in preparations from bovine (13,14), porcine (15) and monkey AP is highly correlated.

Fig. 2 shows that PT reversed the dopaminergic inhibition of basal and forskolin-stimulated prolactin release while also preventing the dopaminergic reduction in forskolin-stimulated cAMP accumulation. Somatostatin, which can reduce cAMP levels in other AP cells types (15), was used as a negative control for the mammotroph, having no effect on prolactin release.

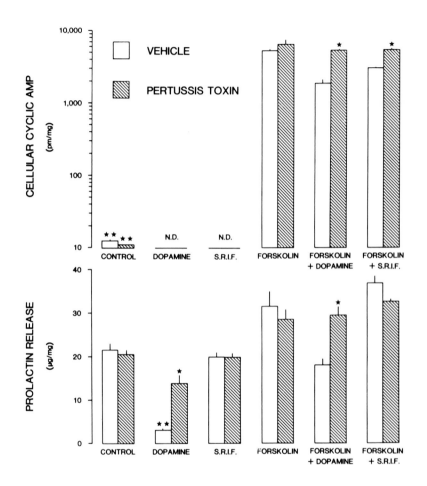

Fig. 2. DA inhibits basal and forskolin-stimulated pro-
lactin release over 4 hr; PT pretreatment reverses this
effect of DA and the DA reduction in cAMP levels. One star
denotes a difference from the respective non-PT treated
control: two stars indicate that the groups are signifi-
cantly different from all other groups. Mean ± SEM; ND =
not determined.

Working with the numerous cell types of the AP in primary culture does not allow one to specify the cell type that initiates a response. This is especially relevant when measuring substances that are probably present in every mammalian cell (e.g., cAMP). The recent application of the hemolytic plaque assay to the AP has brought us one step closer to proving cause and effect in a single cell. Consequently, we identified individual mammotrophs by the erythrocyte hemolytic zones (plaques) developed when incubated with prolactin antibody and guinea pig complement. The results are shown in Fig. 3 and Table I. In brief, DA inhibited the number and size of plaques in both the basal and forskolin-stimulated condition. These effects of DA could be blocked by the DA antagonist spiperone (10 nM, data not shown). Forskolin itself dramaticaly enhanced the number and size of plaques over the vehicle-treated control cells.

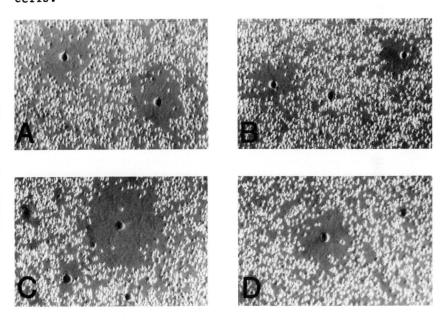

Fig. 3. Micrographs of rat AP cells surrounded by a carpet of erythrocytes. Hemolytic zones around some of the cells indicate the presence of prolactin; the size of the plaque is related to the amount of prolactin released. Plate A = vehicle, Plate B = DA (10 um), Plate C = forskolin (3 uM), Plate D = forskolin + DA. Data from this and 3 other independent studies is summarized in Table 1.

TABLE 1

DA and Forskolin Effects on PRL Plaques in Rat AP Cells

	% Plaques	Area of Plaques [a]
Control	27 ± 1	$1,970 \pm 70$
DA (10 uM)	14 ± 1	$1,130 \pm 60$
Forskolin (3 uM)	35 ± 1	$3,560 \pm 130$
Forskolin + DA	27 ± 1 [b]	$2,590 \pm 100$

a = u^2, all groups different: b = not different from control: mean $\pm$ SEM: 3 independent studies: (400-600 cells scored/slide)

DISCUSSION

The characterization of the AP DA receptor by radioligand binding techniques has identified a site of action for clinically relevant drugs (e.g., bromocriptine) and afforded us the opportunity to define phenomona common to many receptor types (e.g., GTP sensitivity). None of these measurements can specify the partitioning of DA receptors among the various cell types of the AP (e.g., thyrotroph, somatotroph), though it is assumed that the majority of DA receptors reside on mammotrophs. By measuring the impact of DA on PRL release, especially at the level of a single mammotroph (Fig. 3), one can begin to characterize the cell types and subtypes responding to the catecholamine signal.

We have also perturbed several proteins that participate in DA receptor coupling to adenylate cyclase. We demonstrated earlier that DA could inhibit cholera toxin-stimulated cAMP levels and PRL release (11). This bacterial toxin covalently activates the regulatory protein (N_s) linking stimulatory-hormone receptors with catalytic adenylate cyclase (Fig. 4). A similar covalent action on N_i by PT uncouples DA receptor inhibition of cAMP accumulation and PRL release (7). Of interest is the observation that PT continues to extinguish functional DA receptor coupling (i.e., decreased cAMP levels and PRL release), even under cholera toxin- and forskolin-stimulated conditions. Although the precise mechanisms involved remain relatively obscure, there are now known protein targets (Fig. 4) for these various ligands (e.g., DA, PT, cholera toxin, forskolin). Accordingly, isolation of these elements and their use in reconstitution experiments ought to promote a model of the mechanism by which DA inhibits mammotroph adenylate cyclase activity and PRL release.

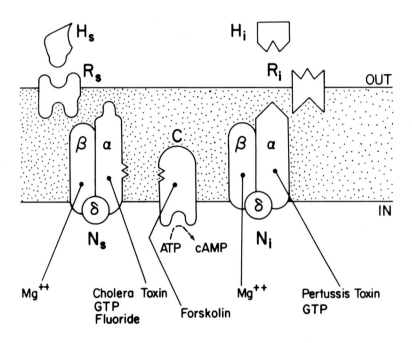

Fig. 4. This model of a mammalian cell surface membrane illustrates the components of hormone stimulated or inhibited adenylate cyclase (AD) activity. Stimulatory (s) and inhibitory (i) hormones (H) and receptors (R) are thought to associate with coupling proteins (N) that regulate the catalytic subunit of AC (C); these coupling proteins are depicted as possible trimers. The proposed site of action of several modulatory agents is also depicted.

REFERENCES

1. Cronin, M.J. and Koritnik, D.R. (1983). *Endocrinology*
    $\underline{112}$, 618-623.
2. DeLean, A., Kilpatrick, B.F. and Caron, M.G. (1982).
    Mol. Pharmacol. $\underline{22}$, 290-297.
3. Kerdelhue, B., Weisman, A.S. and Weiner, R.I. (1981).
    Endocrinology $\underline{109}$, 307-309.
4. Creese, I., Morrow, A.L., Leff, S.E., Sibley, D.R. and
    Hamblin, M.W. (1982). *Int. Rev. Neurobiol.* $\underline{23}$, 255-301.
5. Cronin, M.J. (1982). *In* "Neuroendocrine Perspectives"
    (Eds R.M. MacLeod and E.E. Müller), 1st ed., vol. $\underline{1}$,
    pp. 167-208, Elsevier, New York.
6. Enjalbert, A. and Bockaert, J. (1983). *Mol. Pharmacol.*
    $\underline{23}$, 576-584.
7. Cronin, M.J., Myers, G.A., MacLeod, R.M. and Hewlett,
    E.L. (1983). *Am. J. Physiol.* $\underline{244}$, 499-504.
8. Hewlett, E.L., Cronin, M.J., Moss, J., Anderson, H.,
    Myers, G.A. and R.D. Pearson (1984). *Adv. Cyc. Nucleo-
    tide Res.* $\underline{17}$, 173-182.
9. Seamon, K.B. and Daly, J.W. (1981). *J. Cyc. Nucleotide
    Res.* $\underline{7}$, 201-224.
10. Cronin, M.J., Myers, G.A., MacLeod, R.M. and Hewlett,
    E.L. (1983). *J. Cyc. Nucleotide Res.* $\underline{9}$, 245-258.
11. Cronin, M.J. and Thorner, M.O. (1982). *J. Cyc. Nucleo-
    tide Res.* $\underline{8}$, 267-275.
12. Neill, J.D. and Frawley, L.S. (1983). *Endocrinology*
    $\underline{112}$, 1135-1138.
13. Creese, I. and Snyder, S.H. (1978). *Eur. J. Pharmacol.*
    $\underline{49}$, 201-202.
14. Cronin, M.J. and Weiner, R.I. (1979). *Endocrinology*
    $\underline{104}$, 307-312.
15. Cronin, M.J.(1982). *Life Sci.* $\underline{30}$, 1385-1389.
16. Cronin, M.J., Rogol, A.D., Myers, G.A. and Hewlett, E.L.
    (1983). *Endocrinology* $\underline{113}$, 209-215.

Supported by RCDA1KO4NS500601, NS18408, AM22125, The DuPont
& Rockefeller Foundations and the Pratt Fund.

II. Neuroendocrine Aspects of Neurological Disease

NEUROENDOCRINE CORRELATIONS IN THE CLINIC:
IS THE HYPOTHALAMIC-PITUITARY AXIS THE
WINDOW OF THE BRAIN?

C. Dieguez, J.R. Peters, S.M. Foord, R. Hall,
P.E. Harris and M.F. Scanlon

*Department of Medicine,
Welsh National School of Medicine,
Heath Park,
Cardiff, CF4 4XN, Wales*

INTRODUCTION

It is well known that alterations in pituitary function
occur in widely different pathological situations from
organic brain disease to pituitary disease and primary
target gland disturbances. During the last decade, many
neurohumoral factors have been isolated and characterised
(Table 1), in part because of sophisticated methodological
developments such as HPLC technology. Other methodological
advances such as the developments of more selective drugs
and neurone culture technology have permitted a more satis-
factory chracterisation of neurotransmitter receptor
types. As a consequence of these developments, we have
gained new insights into the regulatory mechanisms involved
in the control of the hypothalamic-pituitary axis. Despite
these advances in understanding, the clinician still faces
major problems when trying to apply such knowledge to
clinical problems. Nevertheless there is no doubt that
diagnostic expertise has been enhanced and hypothalamic
hormone/neurotransmitter therapy is now being used more
rationally and effectively. Not surprisingly, the concept
has emerged of the hypothalamic-pituitary axis as the
"window of the brain", alterations in pituitary control
being representative or typical of a variety of primary
CNS diseases. Whilst this is probably true in general
terms, the many pitfalls associated with interpretation
of data have hindered developments in this area. In this

paper we will summarise the diagnostic and therapeutic advances which have been made over the last decade, while at
the same time highlighting the many problems relating to
in vivo neuropharmacological manipulation and the interpretation of data.

TABLE 1

Anterior pituitary regulators

	Source	NH$_2$Acids	Actions
TRH	1968 porcine ovine	3	↑ TSH, PRL (GH)
LHRH	1969 porcine	10	↑ LH, FSH (GH)
SRIF	1970 ovine	14	↓ GH, TSH
CRF	1981 ovine	41	↑ ACTH (GH)
GRF	1982 pancreas	40,44	↑ GH
Dopamine			↓ PRL, TSH, LH (GH)

PROBLEMS IN THE INTERPRETATION OF IN VIVO DATA

How much information can be gained from the measurement
of circulating anterior pituitary hormone levels, basally or
in response to dynamic testing, about the aetiology, site of
disease or precise neuropeptide/neurotransmitter imbalances
which occur in variety of neuroendocrine and CNS diseases?

Animal versus Human Data

Most of the data regarding the neuroregulation of hypothalamic and pituitary hormones, have been gleaned from studies conducted in rats and there are some fundamental differences compared with primate control mechanisms: for example
oestrogens exert a powerful antidopaminergic action at pituitary level in the rat (1) while they have a facilitatory role
in the dopaminergic inhibition of prolactin release in the
monkey (2). Furthermore, the distribution of several neuroregulators differs between rodents and primates: the greatest
concentrations of LHRH are localized in the preoptic area in
the rat (3) and in the arcuate *nuclei* of primates (4).

Single Neuroregulators with Several Actions

In many instances a single neuroregulator may exert different actions according to its site and target cell: GABA has a stimulatory role in the control of PRL release at central level and an inhibitory action on PRL secretion at the pituitary (5). Moreover, in some instances the same neuroregulator can have opposite actions: dopamine (DA) can produce stimulation or inhibition of PRL secretion *in vitro* depending on the concentration used (6).

Primary Actions versus Compensatory Mechanisms

A single humoral factor is often involved in the neuroregulation of several AP hormones (DA inhibit PRL, TSH and possibly GH secretion at pituitary level (7)). Also AP hormones themselves can modulate the actions of some neuroregulators (PRL increases DA turnover in the hypothalamus (8)). In consequence a similar pattern of response to a particular neuroendocrine test may be detected in several different disease states: similar increases in the TSH response to dopaminergic blockade occur in patients with hyperprolactinaemia (a compensatory mechanism due to the elevated PRL levels feeding back on hypothalamic dopaminergic neurons) and mild hypothyroidism (9). Moreover it is difficult to predict how and when such compensatory mechanisms may operate. Data collected several years ago, which demonstrated that long-term treatment with DA agonists did not lead to hypothyroidism, was interpreted by some to indicate that DA was not involved in the neuroregulation of TSH secretion (10). However it is now well established from both *in vivo* and *in vitro* data that DA does play an inhibitory role in the control of TSH secretion (7) and that the absence of chronic suppression of TSH levels during long-term administration of DA agonists is probably due to a compensatory mechanism, the nature of which is poorly understood at present. In this context, it is relevant to mention recent data which show that after administration of an injectable, slow release preparation of bromocriptine there was a prolonged reduction in basal TSH, T_3 and T_4 levels (11). This suggests that the absence of long lasting suppression of thyroid function during standard oral bromocriptine therapy is of consequence of the shorter plasma half life of this particular preparation.

Measurement of Neuroregulators

   Despite initial hopes, the measurement of hypothalamic
peptides in body fluids and their use as *indices* of hypothalamic function has been largely unrewarding and the method-
ology is fraught with difficulties. The poor sensitivity of
the radioimmunoassays used in relation to the low circulating
concentrations of these peptides has been a major problem.
Furthermore many neuropeptides are also synthesised outside
the CNS and in consequence most of the circulating material
(e.g. TRH and SRIF) is not of neural origin (12). Also the
lack of specific neuropeptide antagonists which could be used
to measure endogenous activities (in an analogous way to the
use of neurotransmitter antagonist drugs) has also hampered
clinical research in this area.

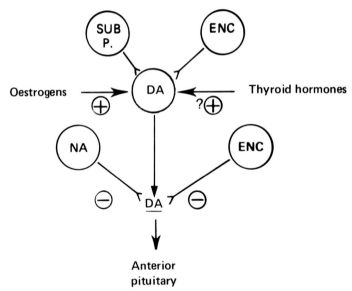

Fig. 1. Regulatory influences on TIDA neurones.

Complex Neuronal Interconnections at All Levels

   The activation of a neuron terminal leading to the subsequent release of a particular neuroregulator is a complex
process involving the participation of many other interneurons
and neuroregulators. A typical schematic outline of this complex interaction is presented in Fig. 1. During activation
of the release of DA from TIDA neuron, many different neuro-

transmitter pathways may be involved in addition to a variety
of peripheral feedback signals (13). Furthermore peripheral
signals may modulate a particular neurotransmitter pathway
via different mechanisms. For example estrogens both stimulate
DA turnover in TIDA neurons (14) and, after conversion to
catechol estrogens (mainly 2-OH-estradiol) may inhibit com-
petitively both tyrosine hydroxylase (15) and catechol-o-meth-
yltransferase (16).

Interaction between Different Neuroregulators

The release of a particular AP hormone is the net result
of the interaction of many stimulatory and inhibitory signals
acting simultaneously on a particular cell. Because of the
large number of signals involved and the several different
mechanisms which may activate a particular signal, it is difficult to assess in the *in vivo* situation which signal may exert
an overriding influence at any given time.

Different Pathways for a Single Neuroregulator

In most instances, a single neurotransmitter or neuropeptide
is involved in the control of several different biological
processes via different pathways. As an example it is believed
that schizophrenic patients have increased dopaminergic tone
at the mesolimbic level. Not surprisingly but to the disap-
pointment of some workers, these patients have normal basal
PRL levels indicating a normally functioning TIDA system (17).

Lack of Specificity of Drugs

A major limitation has been the lack of more selective and
specific drugs which would permit a better understanding of
the different neurotransmitter receptor types and subtypes as
well as providing useful tools for the investigation of neuroendocrine function in the clinic. In particular the lack of
specific serotonin antagonist drugs has led to many erroneous
interpretations of the role of 5-HT in neuroendocrine control
(18). Other drugs which display quite good pharmacological
specificity *in vitro* may produce unexpected actions *in vivo*.
In this context L-dopa, which has been widely used in the study
of neuroendocrine function, is converted to NE as well as DA
and also interacts with 5-HT dependent mechanisms in several
brain areas (19). Therefore we must be very cautious when
trying to decide whether a particular phenomenon observed after
the administration of a given drug is a reliable marker of a
specific biological process.

Alteration in the "Set Point" of Release

An alteration in the negative feedback inhibition of AP hormones leading to a different "set-point" of release is one of the major features of alteration in endocrine control associated with a variety of systemic diseases. For example one of the most widely studied, the "euthyroid sick syndrome", is characterised by low T_3 and T_4 concentrations with normal basal TSH levels and normal TSH responses to TRH suggesting that the lack of increase in TSH levels is due to an alteration in the "set-point" at which the pituitary thyrotroph cells are inhibited by thyroid hormones (19). Quite clearly the interpretation of any data gathered in this situation will be very complex. It is not surprising therefore that in patients with *anorexia nervosa* both enhanced (20) and decreased (21) dopaminergic tone have been postulated as aetiological factors. In consequence opposite therapeutic approaches have been used by several workers (dopamine agonist (22) on the one hand and dopamine antagonists on the other) but with a comparable lack of success in both instances.

TABLE 2

TRH induced GH release

Endocrine	Acromegaly
	Diabetes mellitus
	Hypothyroidism in children
Metabolic	Chronic liver disease
	Chronic renal disease
	Some forms of carcinoma
Neuropsychiatric	Anorexia nervosa
	Schizophrenia
	Depression
	Huntington's chorea
Experimental	*In vitro* cultured pituitocytes
	In vivo rats with ectopically transplanted pituitaries under renal capsule

HYPOTHALAMIC NEUROREGULATORS AND THEIR CLINICAL APPROACHES

The discovery of several of the so-called releasing and inhibiting hormones (RH and IH) has allowed the exploration of new diagnostic and therapeutic approaches to many neuro-endocrine disorders. Here we will review in broad terms the relevance of some of these molecules to diagnosis and therapy.

Thyrotrophin Releasing Hormone (TRH)

Measurement of the TSH response to TRH is of established value in the assessment of thyroid status. It is particularly useful in excluding 1° hyperthyroidism from any cause in the investigation of patients with ophtalmic Grave's disease who do not show the classical features of this disorder and in the detection of subclinical hypothyroidism when basal TSH levels may be high, normal or only marginally elevated.

The TSH response to TRH is also useful as an index of hypo-thalamic-pituitary function but results should be interpreted with caution when distinguishing between pituitary and hypo-thalamic disease. In the rare condition of TSH secreting pituitary adenomas the TSH response to TRH is usually absent in the face of elevated basal TSH and thyroid hormone levels.

Assessment of GH responsiveness to TRH is useful in the detection of altered dynamics GH regulation (Table 2) and, in the case of acromegaly, abolition of the GH release following TRH is a good parameter of successful transpenoidal surgery. In hyperprolactinaemia an absent or reduced PRL response to TRH suggests that presence of a prolactinoma and restoration of PRL responsiveness follows adequate transphenoidal surgery. The clinical value of the measurement of ACTH responses to TRH in Cushing's disease and Nelson's syndrome is yet to be determined.

Despite extensive investigation, the hormonal responses to TRH in various neuropsychiatric disorders are poorly categorised and ill understood. The suppressed TSH responses in depression and paradoxical GH responses in depression, *schizophrenia* and *anorexia nervosa* may well reflect different aetiological sub-types within these groups and could lead to a more rational diagnosis and therapy. Further studies are clearly necessary. After initial enthusiasm it now seems unlikely that TRH itself has any therapeutic value in depression (24).

Gonadotrophin Releasing Hormone (LHRH or GnRH)

The diagnostic value of LHRH is not as great as that of
TRH. An exaggerated gonadotrophin response to LHRH can be
seen in patients with primary hypogonadism from any cause
but the elevated basal values are usually sufficient evidence
for diagnosis. This test cannot discriminate clearly between
hypothalamic and pituitary disease unless it it used in combination with the clomiphene test. In general a negative
clomiphene test combined with a positive LHRH test is sugges-
tive of hypothalamic failure.

However in contrast to its low diagnostic value LHRH and
its superagonist analogues have made a great impact in therapeutic terms in recent years to the treatment of several
diverse disorders. Pulsatile LHRH administration is now being
used in the treatment of "hypothalamic hypogonadism" in order
to restore fertility. LHRH superagonist analogues are now
being evaluated and used in the treatment of such diverse
disorders as precocious puberty, endometriosis, prostatic
cancer and breast carcinoma (25).

Somatostatin

The development of this tetradecapeptide as a therapeutic
agent has been limited by its multiple endocrine/metabolic
actions and by its short plasma½life. Recently however, after
several years of intensive effort, a new analogue (SMS 201-
995, Sandoz) has been developed which has a potent and prolonged inhibitory action on GH release with only a transient
suppression of insulin (26). It is hoped that this molecule
will be of therapeutic benefit in the management of acromegaly.

*Corticotrophin Releasing and Growth Hormone Releasing
Factors (CRF and GRF)*

These recently characterised neuropeptides are currently
being evaluated for diagnostic and therapeutic purposes. Data
available so far indicate that a single CRF test is of little
value in the differentiation of Cushing's disease of pituitary
and non-pituitary origin (27). Similarly administration of GRF
to acromegalic patients results in a wide range of GH responses, from blunted to exaggerated. However it is possible
that a GRF test will be of diagnostic value in the differentiation of hypothalamic *versus* pituitary disease as a cause of
short stature (29) and reports about the longer term of use
of GRF in the treatment of these patients are eagerly awaited.

The use of hypothalamic peptides as diagnostic tools is
helpful in some areas (although less than initially anti-
cipated) but this approach has provided little information
as to the aetiology, site of disease or precise, neuropeptide/
neurotransmitter imbalances which exist in neuroendocrine
disturbances. The prospects are better for their use as therapeutic agents.

Neurotransmitters and their Agonists and Antagonists

During the last 10 years and as a consequence of the development of more specific drugs with fewer side effects, it
has been possible to enhance both our diagnostic and therapeutic approach to many neuroendocrine diseases. The introduction of DA agonist therapy with bromocriptine in hyperprolactinaemia and acromegaly is of major importance and totally changed the management and prospects of patients with
these diseases. Also the introduction of some specific D_2 receptor antagonists (metoclopramide, domperidone) and their
diagnostic use in hyperprolactinaemia has thrown some light
on the nature of the disturbances which may occur in these
patients (30).
The use of agonists and antagonists of other neurotransmitters has been less successful than with the dopaminergic
drugs. Adrenergic agonists and antagonists haven been of
little use in the clinical setting, with the exception of
clonidine as test of GH reserve in children with short stature (31). Likewise the use of serotoninergic compounds has
been of little help. Cyproheptadine, a serotoninergic blocker
(and anti-histaminergic, anticholinergic and antiadrenergic
as well) has been used with varying success in the treatment
of Cushing's disease (32). There are also successful claims
for the use of sodium valproate, a gabaergic agonist, in the
treatment of Nelson's syndrome (33). However any therapeutic
usefulness requires further confirmation in both instances.
Histaminergic (34) and gabaergic (35) drugs have also been
explored as agents for the differential diagnosis of hyperprolactinaemia. Encouraging preliminary results have emerged
about the potential of opiate receptor blockade with naloxone
to restore LH pulsatility (36) but the full usefulness of this
compound in diagnosis and therapy remains to be established.

SUMMARY

Although there have been considerable advances in our
understanding of hypothalamic-pituitary regulatory processes
in recent years, the lack of pharmacological agents with

greater selectivity for different receptor types, together
with the lack of antagonists to the hypothalamic peptides,
has restricted our approach to many clinical neuroendocrine
problems. However the availability of new peptide analogues
and long-acting drugs with fewer side effects has provided
us with some new exciting approaches to the treatment of
several diseases and the future is bright in this regard.

REFERENCES

1. Raymond, V., Beaulieu, M., Labrie F. *et al.* (1978).
   Science 200, 1175-1177.
2. Neill, J.D., Frawley, L.S., Plotsky, P.M. *et al.* (1981).
   Endocrinology 108, 489-494.
3. King, J.C., Tobet, S.A., Snavely, F.L. *et al.* (1982).
   J. Comp. Neurol. 209, 287-300.
4. Bugnon, C., Bloch, B. and Fellman, D.C.R. (1976). *Acad.Sci.*
   282, 1625-1628.
5. Casanueva, F., Apad, J., Locatelli, V. *et al.* (1981).
   Endocrinology 109, 567-575.
6. Denef, C., Manet, D. and Dewals, R. (1980). *Nature* 285,
   243-245.
7. Foord, S., Peters, J.R., Dieguez, C. *et al.* (1983). *Endo-crinology* 112, 1567-1577.
8. Cramer, O.M., Parker, C.R. and Porter, J.C. (1979). *Endo-crinology* 105, 636-643.
9. Peters, J.R., Foord, S., Dieguez, C. *et al.* (1983). *Clin. Endocrinol. Metab.* 12, 669-694.
10. Ranta, T., Mannisto, P. and Tuomisto, J. (1977). *J. Endocr* 72, 329-335.
11. Portman, L., Felber, J.P., Maeder, E. *et al.* (1984). *In* "Proceedings of the 1st ENEA meeting, Basle" Abstract E.4.10.
12. Engler, D., Scanlon, M. and Jackson, I.M. (1981). *J. Clin. Invest.* 67, 800-808.
13. Wass, J.A. (1983). *Clin. Endocrinol. Metab.* 12, 695-724.
14. Moore, K.E., Annunziato, C., Gudelsky, G.A. (1978). *Adv. Biochem. Psychopharmacol.* 19, 193-216.
15. Foreman, H.M. and Porter, J.C. (1980). *J. Neurochem.* 34, 1175-1183.
16. Ball, P., Knuppen, R., Haupt, M. *et al.* (1972). *J. Clin. Endocrinol. Metab.* 34, 736-746.
17. Molitch, M.E. and Hou, S.H. (1983). *Clin. Endocrinol. Metab.* 12, 825-851.
18. Scanlon, M., Rodriguez-Arnao, M.D., Hall, K. *et al.* (1979) *J. Endocrinol. Invest.* 2, 307-331.
19. Jacobs, B.L. (1974). *Psychopharmacologia* 39, 81-90.

20. Barry, V.C., Klawans, H.L. (1976). *J. Neurol. Trans.* **38**, 107-122.
21. Mawson, A.R. (1974). *Psychol. Med.* **4**, 289-308.
22. Harrower, A.D.B., Yap, P.L., Nairn, I. *et al.*(1977). *Br. Med. J.* **2**, 156-159.
23. Mora, B., Hassanyeh, F., Schapira, K. *et al.*(1980). *Proc. Aust. Acad. Sci.* 59-61.
24. Scanlon, M., Peters, J.J.R., Foord, S.*et al.*(1983). *In* "TRH" (Eds E.C. Griffiths and G.W. Bennett), pp.303-314, Raven Press, New York.
25. Sandow, J. (1983). *Clin. Endocrinol.* **18**, 571-592.
26. Plewe, G., Beyer, J., Krause, W. *et al.*(1984).*Lancet* II **84**, 782-784.
27. Orth, D.N., DeGold, C.R., Decherney, G.S. *et al.* (1982). *J. Clin. Endocrinol. Metab.* **55**, 1017-1019.
28. Shibasaki, T., Shizume, K., Masuda, A. *et al.*(1984). *J. Clin. Endocrinol. Metab.* **58**, 215-217.
29. Takano, K., Hizuka, N., Shizume, K. *et al.* (1984). *J. Clin. Endocrinol. Metab.* **58**, 236-241.
30. Peters, J.R., Foord, S., Dieguez, C. *et al.*(1982). *In* "Microprolactinoma" (Ed. G. Molinnatti), pp. 21-34, Excerpta Medica, Amsterdam.
31. Gil, A.D., Topper, E. and Laron, Z. (1979). *Lancet* ii, 278-280.
32. Hsu, T.H., Gann, D.S., Tsan, K.W. *et al.* (1981). *Johns Hopkins Med. J.* **149**, 77-83.
33. Jones, M.T., Gillham, B., Beckford, U. *et al.* (1981). *Lancet* i, 1179-1181.
34. Gonzalez-Villapando, C., Szabo, M., Frohman, L.A. (1980). *J. Clin. Endocrinol. Metab.* **51**, 1417-1424.
35. Melis, C.B., Paoletti, A.M., Mais, V. *et al.* (1982). *J. Clin. Endocrinol. Metab.* **54**, 485-489.
36. Lamberts, S.W.J., Fimmers, J.M., Jong, F.H. (1981). *Fertil. Steril.* **36**, 678-681.

PARATHYROID HORMONE LEVELS IN NORMALS AND PARKINSONIANS AFTER DOPAMINE INFUSION

Peter A. LeWitt, M.D.*, Richard P. Newman, M.D.**,
Donald B. Calne, D.M., F.R.C.P.[+]
Michael O. Thorner, M.B., M.R.C.P.[++]
Michael Wills, M.D., Ph.D.[++]

*Department of Neurology, Lafayette Clinic,
951 E. Lafayette, Detroit, MI 48207 U.S.A.

**Dent Neurologic Institute, Buffalo, N.Y. U.S.A.

[+]Division of Neurology, University of British Columbia
Vancouver, B.C., Canada

[++]Department of Medicine
University of Virginia School of Medicine
Charlottesville, Virginia, U.S.A.

INTRODUCTION

Dopaminergic mechanisms have been demonstrated in the regulation of a variety of behavioral, neuronal, and neuro-endocrine systems (1-4). In this regard, the many roles for dopamine (DA) have served to obscure earlier distinctions between the physiological concepts of "neurotransmitter" and "neuromodulator" (5). The alteration of dopaminergic function is a key factor in the pathophysiology of several neurological and psychiatric disorders, the most common being parkinsonism and schizophrenia. It has become especially clear, from studies with NMPTP, a toxin (6) specific for the dopaminergic nigro-striatal system, that virtually all parkinsonian impairments of motor function can be modeled by a deficiency of nigrostriatal DA. In Parkinson's disease, however, the loss of dopaminergic neurons may extend to other DA systems of the brain (7), just as the biochemical alterations may involve other brain

DOPAMINE AND NEUROENDOCRINE
ACTIVE SUBSTANCES
ISBN 0 12 209045 4

neurotransmitter systems (8,9). The role of these extra-striatal changes in neurotransmitters remains to be explored in the light of impaired cognition and other neuropsychological deficits (10-12) of parkinsonism.

In the current ignorance how Parkinson's disease is initiated and progresses, little is known about systemic features of the disorder. The tendency for seborrhea may be a peripheral manifestation of central autonomic dysregulation, while low blood pressure seen in some (13) but not all (14) parkinsonians may also be derived from the central nervous system. Among a myriad of studies undertaken to find systemic indicators of parkinsonism, only a few have established differences outside the nervous system between parkinsonians and age-matched normals. For example, (^{3}H) spiroperidol binding to blood lymphocytes in untreated parkinsonians was claimed to be decreased in proportion to disability, as contrasted with normals (15). A subsequent study (16) of this non-specific binding confirmed the difference between normals and parkinsonians, although binding did not correlate with clinical symptomatology. Yamaguchi and colleagues (17) have reported that serum biopterin concentrations after oral tyrosine loading showed significantly less of an increase than did levels measured in healthy, age-matched controls. Since the release of prolactin is under inhibitory dopaminergic control by the hypothalamus, one might expect parkinsonians to exhibit higher prolactin levels than normals. However, baseline levels of prolactin, as well as the rise of prolactin induced by thyrotropin-release hormone are normal in parkinsonians (18). The only abnormality to emerge was an attenuation of the prolactin response to TRH in parkinsonians receiving levodopa or bromocriptine.

Dopaminergic neurotransmission takes place both inside and outside of the central nervous system, though the physiological roles of these peripheral systems (apart from neuroendocrine effects) have not been well elucidated. High concentrations of dopamine and its major metabolite, homovanillic acid, are found in peripheral nerves, especially those with autonomic fibers (19). The regulation of renal blood flow appears to be mediated through dopamine receptors linked to adenylate cyclase (20). Features of the latter two peripheral dopaminergic systems have not been compared between parkinsonian and control populations. In this study, we have attempted to determine whether there are abnormalities of regulation of parthyroid hormone in parkinsonian subjects, since the parathyroid glands in some species have been shown to possess D-1 receptors (21). In this regard, we hoped to learn if the vulnerability of dopaminergic systems in the brain extends to other tissues.

In dispersed bovine parathyroid cells, the response to dopamine and compounds with related properties of dopamine agonism are a 2-3 fold increase of parathormone release (22). An *in vivo* confirmation of this effect has been shown by infusing dopamine in cattle (23). Delivery of 0.4 mcg/kg body weight per minute led to a significant rise in parathormone plasma concentration, which rapidly returned to baseline with cessation of the dopamine infusion. In the current study with parkinsonians and normals, we hope to explore whether human parathyroid hormone release is regulated by dopamine.

MATERIALS & METHODS

Five normal subjects (three women, two men, mean age 47.2 years with range 24-57) were controls. Two male parkinsonians, age 60 and 61, were tested. One had never received medications, while the other had been poorly responsive to levodopa plus carbidopa so this medication had been discontinued three months prior to study.

All of the subjects had normal indices of serum calcium, phosphate, and other electrolytes. There was no evidence of bone disease or any endocrine disturbances. All women were post-menopausal.

Design of Study

Each subject was admitted to the hospital and provided informed consent. All were fasted overnight, and received only fruit juice during testing the next day, as desired. A heparin-lock indwelling venous cannula was placed in a forearm vein for drawing blood, while a forearm vein in the opposite arm was used for the infusion of dopamine. For all patients, the first blood sample was obtained at 7 a.m., and subsequently samples were collected at 15 minute intervals from 8 a.m. to 4 p.m. A 0.9% saline infusion commenced at 7 a.m. Dopamine hydrochloride was infused at a constant rate of 4.0 mcg/kg body weight per minute, beginning at 9 a.m. and lasting for a period of 4 hours.

Blood was collected on ice and serum was extracted after centrifugation. Coded samples were stored at −70°C, and the parathyroid hormone level was measured by radioimmunoassay.

RESULTS

During the 9 hours of testing (including the period of dopamine infusion), no significant fluctuation occurred in the serum levels of parathyroid hormone in the control subjects or parkinsonians. Transient nausea was experienced by one patient, but no disturbances of blood pressure or pulse were encountered. The mean values of parathyroid hormone did not correlate to the age or sex of subjects. Although there was a tendency for the two parkinsonians to have lower parathyroid hormone levels, comparison of the two groups by Students t-test yielded no significant difference.

The results of the assays are summarized in Table 1.

TABLE 1

Serum Parathyroid Hormone Levels Averaged from Values Before, During, and After Dopamine Infusion

Normals	ng/ml		S.E.M.
	1.25	±	0.029
	0.77	±	0.080
	0.27	±	0.091
	0.93	±	0.046
	2.76	±	0.075
(mean)	(1.20	±	0.42)
Parkinsonians			
	0.39	±	0.014
	0.33	±	0.0081
(mean)	(0.36	±	0.030)

DISCUSSION

In the 7 subjects, there was little variation in serum parathyroid hormone levels over 9 hours. The parkinsonian subjects did not differ from the normals, and there was no effect from the 4 hours of dopamine infusion. The rate of infusion, which is probably the maximum that can be safely employed, is adequate to cause significant suppression of circulating prolactin levels (24). Our findings are in accord with observations that 30 minutes of dopamine infusion is not followed by change in parathyroid hormone levels (24) and the fact that idiopathic Parkinson's disease is not known to be associated with disturbances of *calcium* or parathyroid hormone metabolism. Although rarely parkinsonian features can be a consequence of pseudo-hypoparathyroidism, the neurological syndrome probably derives from the massive deposition of *calcium* within the basal *ganglia*. If dopamine were an important modulator of parathyroid hormone function, it might be expected that the chronic use of L-DOPA might alter normal patterns of parathormone release. Our results lead us to conclude that the physiological control of human parathyroid hormone is not a dopaminergic system, although it is in other animal species. Whether parkinsonian subjects exhibit any degenerative changes in dopaminergic systems outside of the brain still remains to be learned.

REFERENCES

1. Hornykiewicz, O. (1982). *In* "Movement Disorders" (Eds C.D. Marsden and S. Fahn), pp. 41-58, Butterworth Scientific, Boston.
2. Lancranjan, I. (1981). *J. Neurol. Transm.* 51, 61-82.
3. Goldstein, M., Calne, D.B., Lieberman, A., Thorner, M.O. (Eds)(1980). *In* "Ergot Compounds in Brain Function", Raven Press, New York.
4. Majovski, L.V., Jacques, S., Hartz, G. and Fogwell, L.A. (1981). *Neurosurgery* 9, 751-757.
5. Calne, D.B. (1979). *Neurology* 29, 1517-1521.
6. Burns, R.S., Chieveh, C.C., Markey, S.P. *et al.* (1983). *Proc. Natl. Acad. Sci.* 80, 4546-4550.
7. Javoy-Agid, F., Ruberg, M., Taquet, H., Sudler, J.M. *et al.* (1982). *In* "Gilles de la Tourette Syndrome" (Eds A.J. Friedhoff and T.N. Chase), pp. 151-163. Raven Press, New York.
8. Chase, T.N. (1980). *In* "Neurobiology of Cerebrospinal Fluid" (Ed. J.H. Wood), vol. 1, pp. 207-218, Plenum Press, New York.
9. Fahn, S., Libsch, L.R. and Cutler, R.W. (1971). *J. Neurol. Sci.* 14, 427-455.
10. Boller, F. (1980). *J. Clinical Neuropsych.* 2, 157-172.
11. Pirozzolo, F.J., Hansch, E.C., Mortimer, J.A., Webster, D.D. and Kuskowski, M.A. (1982). *Brain and Cognition* 1, 71-83.
12. Stern, Y., Mayeux, R., Rosen, J. and Ilson, J. (1983). *J. Neurol. Neurosurg. Psychiatr.* 46, 145-151.
13. Barbeau, A. and McDowell, F.H. (Eds)(1970). *In* "L-Dopa and Parkinsonism", F.A. Davis Company, Philadelphia.

14. Aminoff, M.J., Gross, M., Laatz, B., Vakil, S.D. *et al.* (1975). *J. Neurol. Neurosurg. Psychiatr.* 38, 73-77.
15. LeFur, G., Meininger, V., Baulac, M., Phan, T. and Uzan, A. (1981). *Rev. Neurol. (Paris)* 137, 89-96.
16. Maloteux, J.M., Laterre, C.E., Hens, L. and Laduron, P.M. (1983). *J. Neurol. Neurosurg. Psychiatr.* 46, 1146-1148.
17. Yamaguchi, T., Nagatsu, T., Sugimoto, T., Matsuura, S. *et al.* (1983). *Science* 219, 75-77.
18. Eisler, T., Thorner, M.O., MacLeod, R.M., Kaiser, D.L. and Calne, D.B. (1981). *Neurology* 31, 50-55.
19. Lackovic, Z., Kleinman, J., Karoum, F. and Neff, N.H. (1981). *Life Sciences* 29, 917-922.
20. Kebabian, J.W., Petzold, G.L. and Greengard, P. (1972). *Proc. Natl. Acad. Sci.* 69, 2145-2149.
21. Brown, E.M., Attie, M.F., Reen, S., Gardner, D.G., Kebabian, J. and Aurbach, G.D. (1980). *Molec. Pharmacol* 18, 335-340.
22. Brown, E.M., Carroll, R.J. and Aurbach, G.D. (1977). *Proc. Natl. Acad. Sci.* 74, 4210-4213.
23. Blum, J.W., Kunz, P., Fischer, J.A., Binswanger, U. *et al.* (1980). *Am. J. Physiol.* 239, 255-264.
24. Bansal, S., Woolf, P.D., Fischer, J.A. and Caro, J.F. (1982). *J. Clin. Endocrinol. Metab.* 54, 651-652.

CEREBROSPINAL FLUID SOMATOSTATIN-LIKE-IMMUNOREACTIVITY IN RELATION TO CEREBRAL ATROPHY AND DEMENTIA

Erik Dupont*, Stig Engkiaer Christensen+
Per Bo Jørgensen*, Bent de Fine Olivarius* and
Hans Ørskov++

*University Department of Neurology,
+Second University Clinic of Internal Medicine,
++Institute of Experimental Clinical Research,
Aarhus Kommunehospital,
DK-8000 Aarhus C, Denmark

INTRODUCTION

The tetradecapeptide somatostatin was originally isolated and characterized from hypothalamic extracts (1,2). Later, somatostatin-like-immunoreactivity (SLI) was found in abundance in many other areas of the central nervous system: cerebral cortex, basal ganglia and spinal cord (3-6). Like many other neuropeptides somatostatin is found also in the gastrointestinal tract (7-9). Within the central nervous system somatostatin functions as hormone, neurotransmitter and/or synapsemodulator (10-12). Soon after its discovery somatostatin was identified in cerebrospinal fluid (CSF-SLI) (13,14). Measurements on cerebrospinal fluid have made it appearent that some degenerative disorders of the central nervous system are reflected by alterations in CSF-SLI levels (13-19).

We previously reported findings of irreversible low CSF-SLI levels in Parkinson's disease, with values uncorrelated to age, sex, duration of disease, stages of disability, main clinical symptoms and drug treatment (20). This finding may be interpreted either as a consequence of the specific pathophysiological mechanisms of the disease or as an unspecific phenomenon. Reduced CSF-SLI levels have been demonstrated in two disorders both characterized by cerebral atrophy and dementia: presenile and senile dementia of Alzheimer type (18, 19) and Huntington's chorea (17).

DOPAMINE AND NEUROENDOCRINE
ACTIVE SUBSTANCES
ISBN 0 12 209045 4

The aim of the present study was to examine the possible impact on CSF-SLI concentrations of cerebral atrophy and/or dementia due to a variety of different causes.

MATERIALS AND EXPERIMENTAL METHODS

Patients. Fourty neurological patients examined by computed tomography of the brain (CT scan) were studied. Their diagnoses were:

	number
occupational chronic solvent intoxication (21,22)	21
chronic alcoholism	6
idiopathic presenile dementia	5
posttraumatic headache	4
unspecific headache or vertigo	4

The patients were divided into two groups, one group with normal CT scans and one group with cerebral atrophy, diagnosed in accordance with the criteria of Earnest *et al.* (23) and Damasio *et al.* (24). Cases with changes considered to be age-related or with suspect atrophy were not accepted in the study. None of the patients showed signs of focal cerebral lesions on CT scan or in electroencephalographic recordings. No peripheral neurological deficits were revealed at clinical examination.

For socio-economical purposes thirty-two of the patients were psychologically tested for dementia.

Informed consent was obtained from all subjects.

Lumbar puncture. Lumbar puncture was performed in the morning at bedrest after an overnight fast. The 2nd to 4th ml were collected for radioimmunoassay of somatostatin and were immediately mixed with EDTA (final dilution 269 mmol per liter) and frozen until analysis. Specimens appearing blood-stained were discarded.

Chemical analysis. CSF somatostatin was measured by the radioimmunoassay technique, using wick-chromatography for the separation of free and antibody-bound antigen (25). Fifty microliters of antibody (1:1000) were added to 250 μl standard or sample of CSF and incubated for 24 hours at 4°C; then 50 μl of monoiodinated ^{125}I-Tyr^{11}-somatostatin was added and incubated for another 24 hours before separation. Incubation damage, checked in each sample by omitting the antibody, showed neglible denaturation of ^{125}I-Tyr^{11}-somatostatin (26). Determinations were done in triplicate. Intra-assay and interassay coefficients of variation were 5.5% and 10%, respectively; the detection limit was 2 pg per milliliter. Cell

count, determination of total protein, and immunoglobulin
were performed by standard methods.

Values are presented as mean $\pm$ SEM. Differences between
groups were analyzed by Student t test.

RESULTS

Subjects without cerebral atrophy (n = 19) had normal CSF-
SLI levels with a mean of 147.5 $\pm$ 7.8 (pg/ml $\pm$ SEM) (20,28).
The patients with cerebral atrophy (n = 21) had reduced CSF-
SLI concentrations with a mean of 106.0 $\pm$ 3.4 (p < 0.01). Patients with solely cortical cerebral atrophy (n = 14) had
higher CSF-SLI values than patients with cortical as well as
central cerebral atrophy (n = 7), the concentrations being
110.5 $\pm$ 7.7 and 97.3 $\pm$ 9.0, respectively. Patients with cerebral atrophy had higher mean age than those without atrophy:
51.6 $\pm$ 3.1 (years $\pm$ SEM) versus 43.2 $\pm$ 2.4.

The patients with definite dementia (n = 15) had lower
CSF-SLI values than those without dementia (n = 17), the mean
values being 102.9 $\pm$ 6.3 (pg/ml $\pm$ SEM) and 152.0 $\pm$ 11.2, respectively (p < 0.01). Thirteen of the patients with dementia
had cerebral atrophy and two normal CT scans. Of the seventeen patients with no dementia cerebral atrophy was found in
6 and normal CT scans in 11 patients.

DISCUSSION

The results demonstrate an association between cerebral
atrophy and/or dementia and low CSF-SLI concentrations. The
patients examined here had brain affections of different
causes as chronic intoxication by organic solvents, alcohol
abuse and cerebral commotion, or being due to unknown factors. Our finding of low values of CSF-SLI in patients with
cerebral atrophy is in agreement with the observation of
Kohler *et al.* who studied nine patients with marked brain
atrophy (16).

The concept of cerebral atrophy as defined by CT scan is
complex, as it is important to account for age related changes (23). In the present work only cases with definite cortical and/or central cerebral atrophy were included (23,24).
The presence or extent of cerebral atrophy appearing on CT
scan is of limited value in the diagnoses of dementia. This
study confirms that subjects with no intellectual impairment
may show cortical shrinkage and/or ventricular enlargement,
even some demented subjects may show no atrophy on CT scan
(27).

The patients with brain atrophy in the present study were
older than the subjects without atrophy. The age difference,

however, does probably not account for the lowered CSF-SLI
levels in the subjects with atrophy. In previous studies (15,
20,28) we found no correlation between CSF-SLI concentrations
and age, and this is in agreement with Kohler *et al.* (16).

The correlation between cerebral atrophy and/or dementia
and low CSF-SLI values is also demonstrated by the findings
of low values in presenile and senile dementia of Alzheimer
type (18,19) and in Huntington's chorea (17). The low lumbar
CSF-SLI concentrations found in these various conditions probably reflect a reduction of the somatostatin pool and turnover in the atrophic/demented brain (16). Reduced SLI concentrations have been demonstrated in cerebral cortex and
limbic system in Alzheimer dementia (29-32). As the major
amount of the central nervous system somatostatin is contained within the cerebral cortex a correlation between cortical
and CSF-SLI concentrations might be expected (5,6,19). Our
previously reported findings of normal CSF-SLI values in amy-
otrophic lateral sclerosis (20) and benign essential tremor
(28), disorders not associated with cerebral atrophy or dementia, are in agreement with this concept. We have earlier
shown that the major part of CSF-SLI is probably released
diffusely from the brain and spinal cord with no evidence of
leakage into the cerebral ventricles of blood-borne SLI or
of relationship to hypothalamic secretory activity (33). The
small spinal cord pool of SLI (5) cannot account for the substantial decrease in CSF-SLI levels observed in Alzheimer dementia (19).

The earlier finding of irreversible low CSF-SLI values in
Parkinson's disease with low values already from the beginning of clinical symptoms remains unexplained (20). Epelbaum
et al. found SLI concentrations in the frontal cortex significantly reduced in parkinsonian subjects who were slightly
to severely demented, compared to controls and to non-demented parkinsonians. Significant reductions were also demonstrated in the hippocampus and entorhinal cortex of severely
demented subjects (34). Rinne *et al.* found reduced SLI concentrations in the frontal cortex only. The reduction was related to the severity of dementia (32). These cortical changes in SLI concentrations in Parkinson's disease may not explain our finding of low CSF-SLI levels in non-demented parkinsonian patients at the start of clinical symptoms. In
this disease there is a high incidence of cerebral atrophy
already at onset of clinical symptoms (35). Further a high
incidence of cognitive deficits has been demonstrated, even
in presence of normal CT scans (36).

The role(s) of somatostatin in neurotransmission is still
largely unknown. Interactions have been shown between somatostatin and other neurotransmitters (37-39). The growing evi-

dence of Parkinson's disease being a generalized brain disorder, with extensive nigral cell loss as well as other alterations of transmitter functions, seemingly preceeding the appearance of clinical symptoms by months or even years may
explain an early functional or structural impairment of soma-
tostatinergic neurons and low CSF-SLI values (32,40).

REFERENCES

1. Vale, W., Brazeau, P., Grant, G., Nussey, A., Burgus, R.,
    Rivier, J., Ling, N. and Guillemin, R. (1972). *C.R.
    Acad. Sci.* 275, 2913-2916.
2. Brazeau, P., Vale, W., Burgus, R., Ling, N., Butcher, M.,
    Rivier, J. and Guillemin, R. (1973). *Science* 179,
    77-79.
3. Finley, J.W.C., Maderdrut, J.L., Roger, L.J. and Petrusz,
    P. (1981). *Neuroscience* 6, 2173-2192.
4. Hökfelt, T., Johansson, C., Ljungdahl, A., Lundberg, J.M.,
    Schultzberg, M., Fuxe, K., Skerboll, L., Schwarcz, R.
    and Goldstein, M. (1980). *In* "Parkinson's Disease -
    Current Progress, Problems and Management" (Eds U.K.
    Rinne, M. Klingler and G. Stamm), pp. 29-48. Elsevier,
    Amsterdam.
5. Bennett-Clarke, C., Romagnano, M.A. and Joseph, S.A.
    (1980). *Brain Res.* 188, 473-486.
6. Cooper, P.E., Fernstrom, M.H., Rorstad, O.P., Leeman, S.E.
    and Martin, J.B. (1981). *Brain Res.* 218, 219-232.
7. Luft, R., Efendić, S., Hökfelt, T., Johansson, O. and
    Arimura, A. (1974). *Med. Biol.* 52, 428-430.
8. Orci, L., Baetens, D., Ravazzola, M., Malaisse-Lagae, F.,
    Amherdt, M. and Rufener, C. (1976). *In* "Endocrine
    Gut and Pancreas" (Ed. T. Fujita), pp. 73-88. Elsevier,
    Amsterdam.
9. Alumets, J., Sundler, F. and Håkanson, R. (1977). *Cell
    Tiss. Res.* 185, 465-479.
10. Christensen, S.E., Dupont, E., Hansen, Aa.P., Olivarius,
    B. de Fine and Ørskov, H. (1980). *In* "Parkinson's
    Disease - Current Progress, Problems and Management"
    (Eds U.K. Rinne, M. Klingler and G. Stamm), pp. 49-59.
    Elsevier, Amsterdam.
11. Reichlin, S. (1983). *N. Engl. J. Med.* 309, 1495-1501.
12. Reichlin, S. (1983). *N. Engl. J. Med.* 309, 1556-1563.
13. Patel, Y.C., Rao, K. and Reichlin, M.D. (1977). *N. Engl.
    J. Med.* 296, 529-533.
14. Kronheim, S., Berelowitz, M. and Pimstone, B.L. (1977).
    Clin. Endocr. 6, 411-415.

15. Sørensen, K.V., Christensen, S.E., Dupont, E., Hansen,
    Aa.P., Pedersen, B. and Ørskov, H. (1980). *Acta Neurol.*
    Scand. 61, 186-191.
16. Kohler, J., Schroeter, E. and Cramer, H. (1982). *Arch.*
    Psychiatr. Nervenkr. 231, 503-508,
17. Cramer, H., Kohler, J., Oepen, G., Schomburg, G. and
    Schroeter, E. (1981). *J. Neurol.* 225, 183-187.
18. Oram, J.J., Edwardson, J. and Millard, P.H.(1981).
    Gerontology 27, 216-223.
19. Wood, P.L., Etienne, P., Lal, S., Gauthier, S., Cajal, S.
    and Nair, N.P.V. (1982). *Life Sci.* 31, 2073-2079.
20. Dupont, E., Christensen, S.E., Hansen, Aa.P., Olivarius,
    B. de Fine and Ørskov, H. (1982). *Neurology (NY)*
    32, 312-314.
21. Arlien-Søborg, P., Bruhn, P., Gyldensted, C. and Melgaard,
    B. (1979). *Acta Neurol. Scand.* 60, 149-156.
22. Juntunen, J., Hernberg, S., Eistola, P. and Hupli, V.
    (1980). *Eur. Neurol.* 19, 366-375.
23. Earnest, M.P., Heaton, R.K., Wilkinson, W.E. and Manke,
    W.F. (1979). *Neurology* 29, 1138-1143.
24. Damasio, H., Eslinger, P., Damasio, A.R., Rizzo, M., Huang,
    H.K. and Demeter, S. (1983). *Arch. Neurol.* 40, 715-719.
25. Ørskov, H., Thomsen, H.G. and Yde, H. (1968). *Nature* 219,
    193-195.
26. Ørskov, H. and Seyer-Hansen, K. (1974). *Eur. J. Clin.*
    Invest. 4, 207-211.
27. Jacoby, R. and Levy, R. (1980). *J. Royal Soc. Med.* 73,
    366-369.
28. Christensen, S.E., Dupont, E., Mondrup, K., Olivarius, B.
    de Fine and Ørskov, H. (1984). *In* "Advances in
    Neurology" (Eds R.G. Hassler and J.F. Christ), vol. 40,
    pp. 325-331, Raven Press, New York.
29. Davies, P., Katzman, R. and Terry, R.D. (1980). *Nature*
    288, 279-280.
30. Rossor, M.N., Emson, P.C.E., Mountjoy, C.Q., Roth, S.M.
    and Iversen, L.L. (1980). *Neurosci. Lett.* 20, 373-377.
31. Davies, P. and Terry, R.D. (1981). *Neurobiol. Aging* 2,
    9.14.
32. Rinne, U.K., Rinne, J.O., Rinne, J.K., Laakso, K. and
    Lönnberg, P. (1984). *Acta Physiol. Latinoamer.* 34,
    287-299.
33. Sørensen, K.V., Christensen, S.E., Hansen, Aa.P., Inger-
    slev, J., Pedersen, E. and Ørskov, H. (1981). *Neuro-*
    endocrinology 32, 335-338.
34. Epelbaum, J., Ruberg, M., Moyse, E., Javoy-Agid, F., Dubois
    B. and Agid, Y. (1983). *Brain Res.* 278, 376-379.

35. Schneider, E., Fischer, P.-A., Jacobi, P., Becker, H. and
    Hacker, H. (1979). *J. Neurol. Sci.* 42, 187-197.
36. Lees, A.J. and Smith, E. (1983). *Brain* 106, 257-270.
37. Guillemin, R. (1976). *Endocrinology* 99, 1653-1654.
38. Negro-Vilar, A., Ojeda, S.R., Arimura, A. and McCann,
    S.M. (1978). *Life Sci.* 23, 1493-1497.
39. Richardson, S., Hollander, C.S., D'Eletto, E., Greenleaf,
    P.W. and Thaw, C. (1980). *Endocrinology* 107, 122-129.
40. Marsden, C.D. and Parkes, J.D. (1977). *Lancet* I, 345-349.

NEUROENDOCRINE MODIFICATIONS IN PARKINSON DISEASE DURING DA-AGONIST TREATMENT

T. Caraceni, P. Giovannini, G. Scigliano and E. Parati

Department of Neurology, Istituto Neurologico "C. Besta", Via Celoria 11, 20133 Milano, Italy

INTRODUCTION

In accordance with most authors, we have observed that the basal levels of growth hormone (GH)(3, 8, 12, 15), prolactin (PRL)(1, 5, 10, 11, 15) and thyroid-stimulating hormone (TSH) (2, 9, 10, 16-18) in parkinsonian patients do not differ from those of control subjects of equal age and are not modified after chronic treatment with L-dopa and peripheral dopadecarboxylase inhibitor (13, 14).

Our previous experience showed that the release of TSH induced by thyroid-releasing hormone (TRH) in untreated patients was reduced and that this response was restored after chronic treatment with L-dopa and peripheral dopadecarboxylase inhibitor (14). This finding was ascribed to the existence of a reduced dopaminergic tone in the control of TSH, which was blunted by dopaminergic therapy. Another interesting observation was that after chronic treatment with L-dopa and dopadecarboxylase inhibitor, the release of GH induced by a dopaminergic stimulus appeared reduced (13); this would be in agreement with hyposensitivity provoked by chronic treatment with dopaminomimetic drugs.

To verify our previous observations, parkinsonian patients undergoing chronic therapy with direct dopamine-agonists were studied, with particular attention to the dopaminergic mechanism of GH, PRL and TSH secretion. Moreover, it was considered opportune to establish the behaviour of these same hormones in some parkinsonian patients subjected to subchronic treatment with domperidone, a DA-blocking substance that does not pass the blood-brain barrier.

DOPAMINE AND NEUROENDOCRINE
ACTIVE SUBSTANCES
ISBN 0 12 209045 4

MATERIALS AND METHODS

Patients under Chronic Treatment with Dopamine Agonist Drugs

   Eight patients   (6 females and 2 males, aged 41 to 60 years
= mean age 50.6 years) with idiopathic Parkinson's disease
(PD) of 6 months to 10 years duration (mean = 4.1 years)
treated for 1 year with direct dopamine agonist drugs (2
patients with bromocriptine and 6 with lisuride, at median
doses of respectively 57.5 mg and 2.8 mg) were subjected to
the following tests: lisuride, 0.05 mg i.v., with blood samples
taken at -30, 0, 30, 60, 90, 120, 150 and 180 min; TRH, 200
μg i.v., with samples at -30, 0, 30, 45, 60 and 90 min;
insulin tolerance test (ITT), 0.1 U/kg i.v., with samples at
-30, 0, 30, 45, 60, 90 and 120 min.

Patients under Subchronic Domperidone Treatment

   Four parkinsonian patients (3 females and 1 male, with a
mean age of 46 years) not previously treated with dopaminomimetic drugs and affected for 2 years by PD, received domperidone (90 mg/day) for 10 days. Before and after treatment,
the patients were subjected to ITT, lisuride and TRH tests as
described above.
   Blood levels of GH, PRL, TSH, T3 and T4 were estimated
by radioimmunoassay. The results were expressed in absolute
values ± SEM, and statistical significance assessed by means
of Dunnett's t̲ test (4).
   All patients gave informed consent to undergo the tests.
These were performed early in the morning, about 12 h after
the last drug intake in the treated subjects. All patients
remained supine, and blood samples were taken through a catheter placed in the antecubital vein, which was maintained
patent by a slow saline infusion.

RESULTS

GH

   The basal level of GH in patients chronically treated
with direct dopamine agonist drugs did not differ from those
of normal subjects and remained unchanged after treatment
with domperidone (data not shown). The intravenous administration of lisuride in patients chronically treated with
direct dopamine agonists did not provoke any release of GH,
in contrast with that observed in untreated subjects, where
a peak was reached at 90 min (12.9 ± 3.8 ng/ml)(Fig. 1). In

untreated patients, the administration of domperidone did not
significantly modify the GH response to stimulation by lisuride
(Table 1).

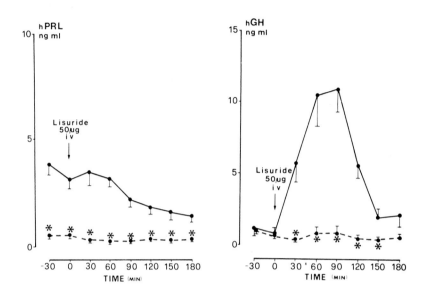

*Fig. 1. PRL and GH responses to lisuride (0.05 mg i.v.) in
8 patients treated with direct dopamine agonist drugs (dotted
line) versus untreated PD subjects (solid line).*

TABLE 1

*GH (ng/ml) response to lisuride (0.05 mg. i.v.) before and
after 10 days of domperidone intake in untreated PD patients.*

| | | \multicolumn{7}{c}{Time (min)} | | | | | | |
		-30	0	30	60	90	120	150
Before	Mean	1.5	0.6	6.6	8.1	10.9	5.5	3.4
	SE	1.0	0.2	1.7	2.1	3.0	1.6	1.3
After	Mean	2.7	0.9	1.2	6.8	6.3	2.0	1.3
	SE	2.0	0.2	0.3	2.4	2.4	0.6	0.3

Administration of insulin to subjects chronically treated
with lisuride or bromocriptine induced a GH release which
was highest at 60 min (peak value 26.2 ± 17.9) and which did
not differ from the response observed in previously untreated
patients (peak value at 60 min 26.2 ± 5.5 ng/ml), before or
after subchronic therapy with domperidone (peak value at 60
min 30.9 ± 4.2 ng/ml)(data not shown).

PRL

   The basal values of PRL were significantly lower in patients treated chronically with direct dopamine agonists than
in untreated patients. These values remained depressed after
the acute administration of lisuride (Fig. 1). The basal
values of PRL after subchronic treatment with domperidone
were significantly ($p<0.001$) elevated with respect to pretreatment values and the administration of lisuride rapidly
induced inhibition of the basal levels, in a manner similar
to that for untreated patients (Table 2).

TABLE 2

*PRL (ng/ml) response to lisuride (0.05 mg i.v.) before and
after 10 days of domperidone treatment in untreated PD patients.*

		\-30	0	30	60	90	120	150
				Time (min)				
Before	Mean	3.3	2.6	3.6	3.4	2.0	1.1	1.3
	SE	0.4	0.3	1.5	0.9	0.8	0.2	0.3
After	Mean	23.2*	20.4*	17.2*	14.9*	12.6*	11.8*	10.8*
	SE	4.9	2.6	2.4	1.3	1.6	0.6	1.5

*P <0.001.

The PRL release induced by TRH was completely blocked in
patients treated with direct dopamine agonists (Table 3). It
should be noted that the basal levels of PRL were always significantly reduced in the group of treated patients with
respect to the untreated patients.

TABLE 3

*PRL (ng/ml) response to TRH in untreated (n=12)
and DA-agonist-treated (n=8) patients*

		-30	0	Time (min) 30	45	60	90
Untreated	Mean	8.0*	7.2*	31.7*	30.8*	28.1*	20.3*
	SE	2.0	1.5	6.2	8.4	8.1	7.6
Treated	Mean	1.9	1.5	2.8	2.4	2.1	1.5
	SE	0.7	0.3	0.6	0.5	0.4	0.2

*p<0.01

TSH

In patients receiving direct dopamine agonists, TRH caused
a TSH release at 30, 45 and 60 min that was significantly
greater than that observed in untreated patients at 30 min
(peak values 9.8 ± 2.3 µU/ml vs 4.5 ± 0.3 µU/ml respectively;
$p < 0.05$). Treatment with domperidone did not appear to modify
the TSH secretory pattern. In all groups the plasma levels
of T3 and T4 were within normal limits.

TABLE 4

*TSH (µU/ml) response to TRH in direct DA-agonist-treated pa-
tients and in PD patients before and after domperidone treatment*

		-30	0	Time (min) 30	45	60	90
DA-agonist-	Mean	2.6	2.5	9.8*	8.5	8.3	6.5
treated	SE	0.2	0.2	2.3	1.2	1.2	0.9
Before	Mean	1.5	1.5	4.5*	4.5	4.1	3.4
domperidone	SE	0.1	0.1	0.3	0.4	0.4	0.5
After	Mean	1.8	1.5	4.5	4.8	4.4	3.5
domperidone	SE	0.3	0.3	1.2	0.5	0.5	0.5

*P<0.05

DISCUSSION

As far as the secretion of PRL is concerned, our results showed: a) a significant reduction in basal levels in subjects undergoing chronic treatment with direct dopamine agonist drugs; b) acute stimulation with lisuride and TRH in the same subjects did not release PRL; c) subchronic treatment with domperidone elevated the basal levels of PRL but did not block the inhibitory effect of lisuride. These data confirm the strong and selective action of direct dopamine agonist drugs in stimulating the dopaminergic receptors controlling PRL secretion and the synthesis of PRL (5).

The normal behavior after subchronic treatment with domperidone did not differ from that recorded with other neuroleptic drugs reflecting normal pituitary function.

The absence of PRL or TSH release in subjects undergoing direct dopamine agonist treatment showed that the secretory mechanisms of both hormones involve dopaminergic modulation and in particular that the DAergic stimulation is a marked inhibitory factor.

As regards to GH, our results show that chronic treatment with direct dopamine agonist drugs does not modify basal levels but blocks the GH release induced by a second dopaminergic stimulant such as lisuride. Since it is known that GH release is under dopaminergic control at hypothalamic level, our data demonstrate that the hypothalamic dopaminergic receptors, which are involved in GH release, find themselves in a condition of hypersensitivity provoked by the pharmacodynamic action of the dopamine agonist drugs. This finding confirms our previous observation of a reduced response of GH to lisuride in patients under chronic treatment with L-Dopa and peripheral dopadecarboxylase inhibitors (6).

Therapy with domperidone, a dopaminergic blocker that does not cross the blood-brain barrier, does not hinder the GH response to lisuride; this finding indirectly confirms that the dopaminergic control of GH is realized centrally.

It is noteworthy that the ITT conserves the capacity to release GH in patients undergoing chronic therapy with direct dopamine agonist drugs. These data (blocked response to lisuride and preserved response to the ITT) demonstrate that the hypoglycemic action does not involve dopaminergic mediation. It is conceivable that the influence of dopaminoagonistic drugs is exerted mainly by modifying the dopaminergic receptor tone.

Finally, of particular interest is the observation of a significant difference in TSH release induced by TRH in subjects undergoing chronic direct dopamine agonist treatment with respect to untreated parkinsonian subjects. In fact, in the latter, the TSH response is reduced, whereas in subjects treated with such drugs it is similar to that of normal subjects. This finding confirms the previous observation of restoration of TSH response in patients chronically treated with L-Dopa (14). The treatment with direct dopaminoagonistic drugs tends to restore the normal response of TSH to TRH and lends support to the possibility of down regulatory mechanisms within the dopaminergic system. In fact, dopaminergic mediation in the release of TSH by TRH is accomplished at hypothalamic level. This is indirectly confirmed by the observation that domperidone does not modify TSH release in our experimental conditions. It is also known that the dopaminergic system interferes with the release of TSH.

The reduced response of TSH to TRH stimulation in untreated patients could reflect an increase in the number of dopaminergic receptors originating from denervation; this is supported by the observation that after treatment with dopaminoagonistic drugs this hyporesponse tends to be corrected.

REFERENCES

1. Bell, R.D., Carruth, A., Rosenberg, R.N. and Boyar, R.M. (1978). *J. Clin. Endocrinol. Metab.* **47**, 807-811.
2. Berger, J.R. and Kelley, R.E. (1981). *Neurology* **31**, 93-95.
3. Boyd, A.E., Lebovitz, H.E. and Feldman, J.M. (1971). *J. Clin. Endocrinol. Metab.* **33**, 829-837.
4. Dunnett, C.W. (1964). *Biometrics* **20**, 482.
5. Eisler, T., Thorner, M.O., MacLeod, R.M., Kaiser, D.L. and Calne, D.B. (1981). *Neurology* **31**, 1356-1359.
6. Falaschi, P., Ruggieri, S., Rocco, A., D'Urso, R., Baldassare, M., Jellamo, R., Conti, L. and Agnoli, A. (1981). *In* "Atti della VII Riunione della Lega Italiana Contro il Morbo di Parkinson" (Eds A. Agnoli and G. Bertolani), pp. 117-126. Guanella, Rome.
7. Galea-Debono, A., Jenner, P., Marsden, C.D., Parkes, J.D., Tarsy, D. and Walters, J. (1977). *J. Neurol. Neurosurg. Psychiat.* **40**, 162-167.
8. Hyyppä, M.T., Langvik, V. and Rinne, U.K. (1978). *J. Neural. Transm.* **42**, 151-157.
9. Kansal, P.C., Buse, J., Talbert, O.R. and Buse, M.G. (1972). *J. Clin. Endocrinol. Metab.* **34**, 99-105.
10. Lavin, P.J.M., Gadwell, M.J., Das, P.K., Alaghband-Zadeh, J. and Rose, F.C. (1981). *Arch. Neurol.* **38**, 759-760.
11. Lawton, N.F. and MacDermot, J. (1980). *J. Neurol. Neurosurg. Psychiat.* **43**, 1012-1015.
12. Lundberg, P.O. (1972). *Acta Neurol. Scand.* **48**, 427-432.
13. Martinez-Campos, A., Giovannini, P., Parati, E., Novelli, A., Caraceni, T. and Müller, E.E. (1981). *J. Neurol.*

Neurosurg. Psychiat. <u>44</u>, 1116-1123.

14. Martinez-Campos, A., Giovannini, P., Novelli, A.,
    Cocchi, D., Caraceni, T. and Müller, E.E. (1982).
    Acta Endocrinol. (Kbh) <u>99</u>, 344-351.

15. Polleri, A., Carolei, A., Rolandi, E., Masturzo, P.,
    Meco, G. and Agnoli, A. (1977). *Neurcpsychobiology*
    <u>3</u>, 42-48.

16. Rabey, J.M., Vardi, Y., Ravid, R. and Ayalon, D. (1981).
    Hormone Res. <u>15</u>, 78-87.

17. Splauding, S.W., Burrow, G.N., Donabedian, R. and Van
    Woert, M. (1972). *J. Clin. Endocrinol. Metab.* <u>35</u>,
    182-185.

18. Wingert, T.D. and Hershman, J.M. (1979). *Neurology* <u>29</u>,
    1073-1074.

DOPAMINE RECEPTOR FUNCTION IN PARKINSON'S DISEASE IN VIVO STUDIES WITH PROLACTIN RESPONSES

A. Laihinen and U.K. Rinne

Department of Neurology, University of Turku, SF-20520 Turku 52, Finland

INTRODUCTION

In Parkinson's disease (PD), progressive destruction of dopamine (DA) neurons occurs in the *substantia nigra*, a process which represents the presynaptic pathology of the disease. On the other hand, it has recently been observed (1-4) that post-synaptic structures are also involved in the pathogenesis of PD, namely changes in the DA receptors in the *striatum*. Prolactin (PRL) secretion is an indicator of the DA receptor function in the pituitary. The hypothalamus has also been shown (5) to be involved in PD.

Del Pozo *et al.* (6) showed that a single 4mg dose of bromo-criptine (BCT) lowered serum PRL for at least 12 hours in normal subjects. Eisler *et al.* (7) found that in PD the resting levels of PRL and the TRH-induced rise in PRL were normal. Levodopa elicited a normal suppression of PRL concentrations in untreated parkinsonian subjects, in whom the major pathological finding was the reduced response to TRH following administration of BCT or levodopa combined with carbidopa.

In the present study, the aim was to investigate the DA receptor function and its relationship to the daily fluctuations in disability of parkinsonian patients by using PRL responses to TRH after BCT pretreatment as an index of DA receptor function.

MATERIALS AND EXPERIMENTAL METHODS

The total number of parkinsonian patients studies was 50, of whom 36 had PD of recent onset (levodopa-untreated) and 14 were advanced parkinsonian patients (levodopa-treated). The control comprised 15 age- and sex-matched subjects. The pa-

tients of recent onset consisted of parkinsonian cases who
were taken to the Department of Neurology for pretreatment
examination. The patients with long-term levodopa treatment
were taken from the follow-up material of parkinsonian out-
patient clinic of the Department.

PRL secretion was tested with a BCT/TRH test. After having
been awake and at rest for one our, the patients were given
1.25 mg of BCT (Parlodel[R]) orally at 8 a.m. Two hours after
this BCT pretreatment, 200 µg of TRH (Inithyran[R]) was given
intravenously to elicit PRL secretion without involvement of
DAergic mechanisms. This procedure made it possible to show
how sensitively the DA receptors on the cell surface of the
lactotrophs reacted to the DA agonist BCT. Plasma PRL concentrations were assayed with a RIA technique (PROL-RIA[R], Insti-
tut des Radioéléments, Belgium).

RESULTS

There was no significant differences between the patient
groups concerning baseline PRL values. In all groups the mean
PRL concentration was well within normal limits. A BCT dose
of 1.25 mg induced PRL suppression both in patients with recent onset PD and advanced parkinsonian patients.

TABLE 1

*Effect of TRH (200 ug I.V.) on prolactin secretion (ug/l)
after BCT pretreatment (1.25 mg by mouth). Mean ± SEM. BCT
given at 0', TRH at 2 h. Basal value taken at 0'.*

Group	n	Basal value	2 h	2 h 20'	3 h
Controls	15	6.9±1.6	4.4±1.2	10.7±2.5	6.7±1.9
Recent onset	36	6.2±0.7	2.9±0.5	5.6±0.7*	3.7±0.6
Advanced/ fluctuations in disability	6	6.8±0.7	3.9±2.5	16.1±5.5**	9.3±3.5
Advanced/ without fluc- tuation	8	8.1±1.8	3.9±0.9	9.0±1.6	6.2±0.8

 * p<0.01 as compared with controls
** p<0.05 as compared with all other groups

According to Table 1, the THR-induced PRL peak was lower (p<0.01) in the patients with PD of recent onset compared with the controls. In the advanced parkinsonian patients suffering from daily fluctuations in disability, the PRL secretion was higher (p<0.05) than in any of the other groups. On the other hand, among advanced parkinsonian patients showing no fluctuations the PRL response to TRH was almost the same as in the control group.

DISCUSSION

The results presented here support the view (7) that PRL responses are sufficiently sensitive to study pituitary DA receptor function *in vivo* in parkinsonian patients. The present findings may be compared with *post mortem* DA receptor studies (1-4,8), according to which most of the parkinsonian patients without levodopa treatment show an increased binding of ^{3}H-spiroperidol in the caudate *nucleus* and *putamen*. In the *striata* of patients who had received levodopa treatment binding studies with ^{3}H-spiroperidol show that the density of D-2 sites is either normal or low. In agreement with these binding results the present findings obtained with PRL responses imply that there is DA receptor supersensitivity in recent onset patients untreated with levodopa, whereas advanced parkinsonian patients show DA receptor desensitization and/or loss of DA receptors if they have daily fluctuations in disability. Apparently, the pituitary DA receptor function is within the normal range in levodopa-treated patients with advanced PD who do not have daily fluctuations in disability.

Furthermore, the present data suggest that the pathological processes in PD are not only localized to the nigrostriatal dopamine neurons but also extrastriatal systems including the hypothalamo-pituitary axis are involved.

ACKNOWLEDGEMENTS

This study was supported by a grant from the Sigrid Jusélius Foundation, Finland.

REFERENCES

1. Reisine, T.D., Fields, J.Z., Yamamura, H.I., Bird, E.D., Spokes, E., Schreiner, P.S. and Enna, S.J. (1977). *Life Sci.* 21, 335-344.
2. Lee, T., Seeman, P., Rajput, A., Farley, I.J. and Hornykiewicz, O. (1978). *Nature* 273, 59-61.

3. Rinne, U.K., Sonninen, V. and Laaksonen, H. (1979). *Adv. Neurol.* <u>24</u>, 259-274.
4. Rinne, U.K., Koskinen, V. and Lönnberg, P. (1980). *In* "Parkinson's Disease, Current Progress, Problems and Management" (Eds U.K. Rinne, M. Klingler and G. Stamm), pp. 93-119, Elsevier, Amsterdam.
5. Langston, J.W. and Forno, L.S. (1978). *Ann. Neurol.* <u>3</u>, 129-133.
6. Del Pozo, E., Brun del Re, R., Varga, L. and Friesen, H. (1972). *J. Clin. Endocrinol. Metab.* <u>35</u>, 768-771.
7. Eisler, T., Thorner, M.D., MacLeod, R.M., Kaiser, D.L. and Calne, D.B. (1981). *Neurology* <u>31</u>, 1356-1359.
8. Rinne, U.K., Rinne, J.O., Rinne, J.K., Laakso, K., Laihinen, A. and Lönnberg, P. (1983). *J. Neural Transm.* Suppl. <u>18</u>, 279-286.

III. Prolactin and Dopamine Agonists

THE PROLACTIN RECEPTOR: LOCALIZATION, AFFINITY LABELLING AND THE IDENTIFICATION OF MONOCLONAL ANTIBODIES

Paul A. Kelly*, Masao Katoh* and Jean Djiane[+]

Laboratory of Molecular Endocrinology, Royal Victoria Hospital, Montreal, Quebec, H3A 1A1, Canada.

[+]*Laboratoire de Physiologie de la Lactation, I.N.R.A., 78350 Jouy-en-Josas, France.*

INTRODUCTION

The primary action of the anterior pituitary hormone prolactin (PRL) is the development of the mammary gland and lactation. In a number of species, however, prolactin has been shown to have other reproductive functions and it is especially important in the regulation of water and ion fluxes in lower vertebrates (1).

Prolactin acts by first interacting with specific receptor sites located at the periphery of the cell. Following binding to the plasma membrane receptor, various effects can be observed including, at the nuclear level, the stimulation of mitotic activity and gene activation; within the cytoplasm, the transcriptional products (mRNA) may be stabilized, translation of the messages occurs, and enzyme systems may be either turned on or off (2).

A great deal of work on the mechanism of prolactin action has utilized the mammary gland as a model. However, PRL receptors can be localized in a number of known target tissues. Once the receptors are localized, it is important to characterize the receptor molecules, and this can best be done by affinity labelling the binding subunit and by production of monoclonal antibodies, which are specific to various domains of the receptor molecule.

MATERIALS AND EXPERIMENTAL METHODS

The localization of PRL receptors was determined in various tissues and species as listed in the RESULTS section. Localization was by immunocytochemistry, radioautography and radioreceptor assay, using [^{125}I] ovine production (oPRL) as labelled ligand (3,4).

Affinity labelling of the PRL receptor was performed using [^{125}I] oPRL bound to receptors and the hormone receptor complex exposed to the photoactive cross-linker N-hydroxy-succinimidyl-4-azidobenzoate (HSAB) for 15 minutes under an ultraviolet light. The molecular weight of the receptor subunit was estimated by SDS polyacrilamide gel electrophoresis of the reaction mixtures in a slab gel, and autoradiography of the dried gels (5,6).

Prolactin receptors were partially purified (7), based on the original procedure described by Shiu and Friesen (8). Polyclonal antibodies to the purified receptors were prepared, which were shown not only to inhibit binding, but also to posess stimulating or inhibiting effects dependent upon the dose of antiserum utilized (2,9,10). Although these antibodies have proven useful, the development of monoclonal antibodies (mAb) to the PRL receptor would allow a number of interesting studies to be done. These include advances in the area of the structure of the receptor molecule, biosynthesis of the receptor, isolation of its mRNA and cloning of a cDNA, and the ultimate purification and structural determination of the receptor and its subunits.

Monoclonal antibodies were produced by conventional approaches by immunizing mice with partially purified PRL receptor for 10 weeks (10 ug every three weeks). Lymphocytes from the spleens of the mice were hybridized with a SP-2 lymphoma cell line (11). Positive hybrides were screened with the ELISA assay using purified receptor and by inhibition of binding.

RESULTS

Localization

Prolactin receptors have been localized in a number of tissues including mammary gland, mammary tumor, liver, kidney, adrenal, ovary, testis, prostate, seminal vesicle, pancreatic islets, lymphoid tissue, pineal body, hypothalamus and choroid plexus (2,12).

Prolactin binding in the brain was first reported by Walsh et al (13) to be localized on ependyma of the rat choroid plexus. Subsequently, Dubé et al (4) confirmed their observations and suggested other possible sites. More recently, Walsh described that following in vivo administration of [^{125}I] oPRL to rats, initial binding occurred at the basal and lateral plasmalemma of the epithel-

ial cells. With time, the radioactive grains in the elec-
tion microscopic autoradiographs were localized over the
interior of the cells in non-lysosomal cytoplasmic organ-
elles (14).

Affinity Labelling of the Receptor

    The effect of increasing concentrations of HSAB on the
affinity labelling of rabbit mammary gland microsomal proteins with (^{125}I) oPRL is shown in Fig. 1. As can be seen,
a single band at M_r=32,000 is observed. The only effect
of increasing the HSAB concentration is to increase non-
specific background. The molecular weight (MW) of the binding component was calculated as the difference in the MW of
the PRL-receptor complex and that of PRL under the conditions of the SDS gel electrophoresis.

(A)   (B)

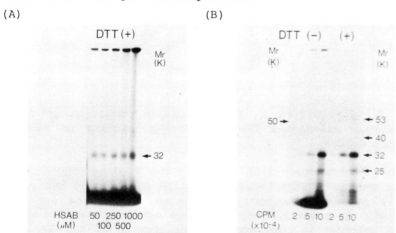

*Fig. 1. (A) Autoradiogram of the effect on increasing con-
centrations of HSAB on the affinity labelling of mammary
PRL receptors. (B) Autoradiogram of (^{125}I) labelled (by
chloramine-T) purified PRL receptors. Electrophoresis was
performed in a 7.5% homogeneous (A) or a 9-15% gradient gel
(B).*

    When a partially purified PRL receptor preparation was
iodinated and analyzed by SDS gel electrophoresis and autoradiography, a similar M_r=32,000 band was the most intense
(Fig. 1, B). Other faint bands were observed, but the majority of the labelled material migrated in the gel in a similar fashion to the major binding subunit of the PRL receptor, as determined by affinity labelling (2, 6).

Monoclonal Antibodies to the Receptor

The ability of four monoclonal antibodies against the prolactin receptor to inhibit [^{125}I] oPRL binding to mammary membranes is shown in Fig. 2.

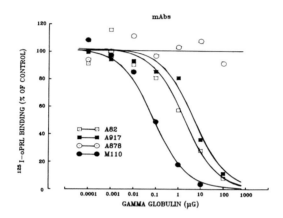

Fig. 2   *Competition by gamma globulin fractions of four monoclonal antibodies for [^{125}I] oPRL binding to rabbit mammary tissue.*

Three of the four mAbs inhibited the binding completely, while another (A878), which was ELISA positive to the partially purified receptor preparation, failed to inhibit binding. Such antibodies, which are not site specific will be of interest in identifying other domains of the PRL receptor.

The binding of [^{125}I] monoclonal antibody (M110) or [^{125}I] oPRL to various tissues from rabbit, rat, pig and a human breast cancer cell line (T47-D) is depicted in Fig. 3. There is good agreement between oPRL and mAb binding in rabbit tissues, but rat tissues, which bind [^{125}I] PRL, do not bind the mAb. Interestingly, mammary tissue from a lactating pig also binds [^{125}I] mAb. This suggests that the binding domains of the receptors from the two species are similar. In fact, the affinity of the mAb for the receptor site is slightly greater than for PRL itself (data not shown). The human breast cancer cell line T47-D possess PRL receptors, as measured by the binding of [^{125}I] hGH, which binds with high affinity to PRL receptors. However, the mAb does not recognize human PRL receptors.

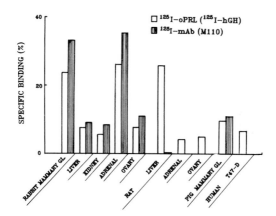

Fig. 3   Specific binding of $[^{125}I]$ labelled oPRL (or hGH) and mAb to PRL receptors from rabbit, rat, pig and human.

The high affinity of mAb M110 for the receptor can be seen in Fig. 4.   The polyclonal antibody produced in a sheep (#151) has been described as being the most potent inhibitor of PRL binding (2,9,10).   The mAb is more than 80-fold more potent in inhibiting PRL binding than the polyclonal antibody.   Ascites fluid from control, non-immunized mice had no effect on PRL binding.

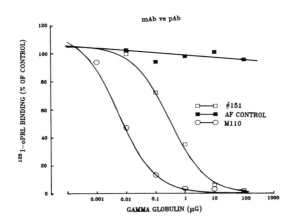

Fig. 4   Comparison of polyclonal (pAb) and monoclonal (mAb) antibodies to inhibit PRL binding to rabbit PRL receptors. A gamma globulin fraction of the pAb (151) or mAb (M110), which was amplified in ascites fluid (AF), as well as an AF control, are included.

The specificity of (^{125}I) mAb binding to rabbit mammary tissues is shown in Fig. 5. All lactogenic hormones compete for the binding site occupied by the labelled mAb, whereas the non-lactogenic hormones oLH, oFSH, oGH and insulin have no effect. Rabbit PRL (rbPRL), which binds with a very poor affinity to rabbit PRL receptors, is also much less capable of inhibiting mAb binding to the PRL receptor.

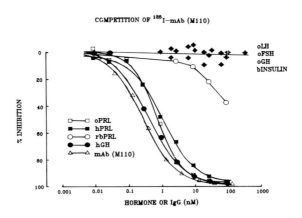

Fig. 5 Specificity of binding of [^{125}I] mAb to rabbit mammary tissue.

DISCUSSION

Prolactin receptors can be localized in numerous tissues, including some within the nervous system. There is an obvious role for PRL receptors in areas such as the hypothalamus to act as a site for short-loop feed back of PRL. The role of PRL receptors in the choroid plexus is as yet unclear. They may serve as a means of transporting PRL through the epithelial cells into the cerebrospinal fluid (CSF), or PRL may have some direct role on the cells of the choroid plexus where CSF is produced.

Our current knowledge of the structure of the PRL receptor is limited. The present data indicate that the major binding component in the membrane of rabbit mammary tissue has a relative molecular mass of 32,000 when affinity labelling techniques combined with SDS-polyacrylamide gel electrophoresis were employed. The M_r = 32,000 binding component does not appear to bind to itself or other binding components through disulfide or other linkages, as dithio-

thretol (DTT) treatment of the cross-linked receptor did
not result in any significant change in the migration of
the hormone-receptor complex (2,6), in contrast to what has
been reported for the insulin receptor, which consists of
four subunits linked by S-S bonds (15,16). The structure
of the PRL receptor in rabbit mammary glands may be more
similar to that of insulin-like growth factor II (17).
Certainly, the relative samll size of the binding subunit
(32K) is in agreement with affinity labelling data of the
PRL receptor in the rat liver (18). All of these receptors
have been reported to be a single binding component.

Monoclonal antibodies to PRL receptors of rabbit mammary
tissue have been produced which have varying specificity.
Some are site-specific and characterization of one (M110)
has demonstrated that it competes for the specific binding
site of PRL and has a slightly higher affinity for that
site than does PRL itself. Specificity studies confirm
that it is indeed specific for lactogenic receptors from
rabbits and at least one tissue from a pig, suggesting a
close similarity of the binding subunit from these two
species. The mAbs which cross-reacted in the ELISA assay,
but not in the binding inhibition assay, are of interest,
as they will allow binding of the hormone and the mAb to
the receptor and subsequentimmunoprecipitation of the complex. These mAbs are currently being characterized.

The monoclonal antibodies which have been produced will
be utilized for immunological localization of receptors in
various target cells. This will greatly increase our knowledge of the fate of receptors following internalization of
the hormone-receptor complex. In addition, specific immu-
noassays for receptors can be developed. Monoclonal antibodies will also be of interest in elucidating the structure of the receptor, studying its biosynthesis, isolating
a mRNA and cloning a cDNA for the receptor protein.

ACKNOWLEDGEMENTS

The authors wish to express their gratitude to Mr. J.
Zachwieja for his excellent technical assistance and Ms.
Diane Déziel for typing the manuscript. The contribution
of the National Hormone and Pituitary Program for providing
hormones is greatly appreciated. These studies were supported by grants from the National Cancer Institute (Canada), Medical Research Council (Canada) and the United
States Public Health Service.

REFERENCES

1. Nicoll, C.S. and Bern, H.A. (1972). *In* "Lactogenic
    Hormones" (Eds G.E.W. Wolstenholme and J. Knight),
    pp. 299-374. Churchill-Livingston, London.
2. Kelly, P.A., Djiane, J., Katoh, M., Ferland, L.H.,
    Houdebine, L.M., Teyssot, B. and Dussanter-Fourt, I.
    (1984). *Recent Prog. Hor. Res.* 40, 379-439.
3. Posner, B.I., Kelly, P.A., Shiu, R.P.C. and Friesen, H.G.
    (1974). *Endocrinology* 96, 521-531.
4. Dubé, D., Kelly, P.A. and Pelletier, G. (1980). *Mol.
    Cell. Endocrinol.* 18, 109-122.
5. Johnson, G.L., MacAndrew, V.I. and Pilch, P.F. (1981).
    Proc. Natl. Acad. Sci. USA 78, 875-878.
6. Kelly, P.A., Katoh, M., Djiane, J. and Sakai, S. (1984).
    Methods in Enzymology (in press).
7. Katoh, M., Djiane, J., Leblanc, G. and Kelly, P.A. (1984).
    Mol. Cell. Endocrinol. 34, 191-200.
8. Shiu, R.P.C. and Friesen, H.G. (1974). *J. Biol. Chem.*
    249, 7902-7911.
9. Djiane, J., Houdebine, L.M. and Kelly, P.A. (1981).
    Proc. Natl. Acad. Sci. USA 78, 7445-7448.
10. Kelly, P.A., Katoh, M., Djiane, J., Houdebine, L.M.,
    Dussanter-Fourt, I. and Teyssot, B. (1984). *Methods
    in Enzymology* (in press).
11. Eisenbarth, G.S. and Jackson, R.A. (1982). *Endocrine
    Rev.* 3, 26-39.
12. Posner, B.I. and Khan, M.N. (1983). *In* "Prolactin and
    Prolactinomas" (Eds G. Tolis, C. Stefanis, J. Mounto-
    kalakis and F. Labrie), pp. 9-18. Raven Press, New
    York.
13. Walsh, R.J., Posner, B.I., Kopriwa, B.M. and Brawer, J.R.
    (1978). *Science* 201, 1041-1043.
14. Walsh, R.J., Posner, B.I. and Patel, B. (1984). *Endo-
    crinology* 114, 1496-1505.
15. Pilch, P.F. and Czech, M.P. (1979). *J. Biol. Chem.* 225,
    1722-1731.
16. Massagué, J., Pilch, P.F. and Czech, M.P. (1980).
    Proc. Natl. Acad. Sci. USA 77, 7137-7141.
17. Massagué, J., Guillette, B.J. and Czech, M.P. (1981).
    J. Biol. Chem. 256, 2122-2125.
18. Borst, D.W. and Sayare, M. (1982). *Biochem. Biophys.
    Res. Commun.* 105, 194-201.

TREATMENT OF PROLACTINOMAS

K. von Werder*, R. Landgraf*, R. Oeckler[+] and H.K. Rjosk[++]

*Medizinische Klinik Innenstadt

[+]Neurochirurgische Klinik Grosshadern

[++]Frauenklinik, University of Munich, 8000 Munich 2, FRG

INTRODUCTION

Hyperprolactinemia, the most common hypothalamic-pituitary disorder in man, may be caused by three different mechanisms (1).

1. Autonomous prolactin (PRL) secretion by a pituitary adenoma (prolactinoma);
2. Reduced or absent dopamine effect on the lactotroph cell;
3. Excessive stimulation of the lactotroph cell overriding physiologic inhibition.

All hyperprolactinemic patients in whom drug induced elevation of PRL-levels, renal failure or hypothyroidism has been excluded harbour most likely a prolactinoma. The latter is supported by the findings of Jung *et al.* (2) who demonstrated microadenomas with high resolution CT in 15 out of 16 hyperprolactinemic women with a normal or equivocal radiological sella.

Though there may be patients with what is called functional hyperprolactinemia, we are still unable to make the differential diagnosis between those two entities (3). For clinical purposes the latter is not very important since the management of both clinical situations is identical.

SPONTANEOUS DEVELOPMENT OF HYPERPROLACTINEMIA

There is very little difference in morphology of small adenomas and invasive macroprolactinomas (4). However, the

spontaneous clinical course may be very different, which has
to be considered in the management of these patients. Thus,
the majority of patients with hyperprolactinemia and a normal
sella turcica or proven microprolactinoma have PRL-levels
which remain within the same range over an observation period
of up to 10 years (5). This is in obvious contrast to the
development of large invasive macroprolactinomas where there
is often only a short history of hyperprolactinemia-related
symptoms (1).

MEDICAL THERAPY OF PROLACTINOMAS

Treatment with Ergot Derivatives

Ergot derivatives with long lasting dopaminergic activity
have been used for the treatment of hyperprolactinemia. The
largest experience has been obtained with bromocriptine which
belongs to the lysergic acid amides and contains a tripeptide
moiety (1). Lisuride and mesulergin (CU 32-085) belong to
the 8α-aminoergoline family whereas pergolide, a very potent
PRL inhibitor, belongs to the clavine family. All these substances lead to dopamine receptor stimulation an inhibition
of PRL-secretion without the uterotonic and vascular effects
found in other ergot alkaloids (1).
Moderately elevated PRL-levels in patients with a normal
sella turcica or a radiologically apparent microprolactinoma
are usually normalized with moderate DA-agonist dosages (1,5).
Though the PRL-lowering efficacy of DA-agonists can be even
more pronounced in patients with extremely elevated PRL-levels (5), these will not always return to normal if they are
above 1000 ng/ml, even if bromocriptine dosages of up to 40
mg and more per day are used (1,5). This great variability
of the responsiveness of PRL-secretion to dopaminergic suppression is also demonstrated during acute dopamine infusion
(6).
Evidence has been presented that the addition of tamoxifen,
an estrogen antagonist, may improve the responsiveness to
bromocriptine in selected cases (7).
In addition to normalization of PRL-secretion, reduction
of tumor mass is an important therapeutic goal in patients
with macroprolactinomas. Since it has been shown that DA-
agonists may lead to dramatic reduction of tumor volume in
the majority of patients with macroprolactinomas (8,9,10,11),
primary medical therapy has become generally accepted in such
patients.

Adenoma Shrinking Effect of DA-Agonists

Eight years ago reports describing reduction of adenoma size after bromocriptine therapy as documented by conventional X-ray were published (for review see 1,5). The tumor-shrinking effect of DA-agonists in humans became more obvious when the regression of suprasellar extension of pituitary macroprolactinomas could be shown by CT (8). DA-agonist induced tumor reduction may occur within days (12).

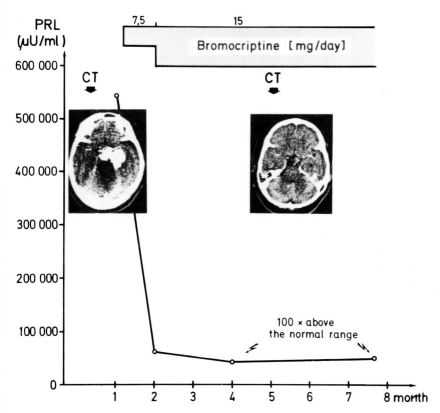

Fig. 1. Disappearance of suprasellar prolactinoma extension during bromocriptine therapy without normalization of PRL-levels. Though PRL-levels remain around 50,000 μU/ml during therapy (upper normal range 500 μU/ml) there is dramatic reduction of supra- and parasellar tumor extension documented by CT-scan during bromocriptine treatment.

Initially, the rapidity of the tumor shrinkage suggested that
tumor apoplexy may be responsible for this phenomenon. However, it could be shown that bromocriptine causes a reduction
of lactotroph cell volume and cytoplasmic structures responsible for prolactin synthesis (13,14). Whether the morpho-
metrically demonstrated diminution in cell volume is the only
mechanism of tumor shrinkage is still uncertain, since a decrease in cell size was also observed in those patients who
had no demonstrable adenoma reduction (15). It would explain
however, that prolactinomas can reexpand after DA-agonist withdrawal and shrink again after re-institution of DA-therapy in
a rapid fashion (13) which could not be accounted for by a
cytotoxic effect of these compounds.However, persisting suppression of PRL-secretion after longterm treatment with dopamine agonists has been observed (16). Recently, Winkelmann
et al. reported permanent normalization of PRL-levels in patients with lactoprolactinomas after withdrawal of longterm
bormocriptine treatment (17). Adenoma shrinkage is also observed in those patients in whom PRL-secretion has not normalized during DA-agonist therapy (Fig. 1.).On the other hand
even complete normalization of PRL-levels in patients with
macroprolactinomas does not imply changes of adenoma volume
(18). Several series have been published reporting the outcome of primary medical therapy of macroprolactinomas (8,9,10,
11), demonstrating that between 50 and 80% of all patients
with macroprolactinomas will respond to DA-agonist therapy
with adenoma shrinkage.However, until now it cannot be predicted which patient will or will not benefit from medical ther
apy concerning the adenoma volume.

The recent report that DA-agonist therapy of longer duration may jeopardize the outcome of later neurosurgical intervention (19) has not been confirmed (20). Prolactinomas very
rarely proliferate during DA-agonist therapy (21). We have
observed one female patient who, after neurosurgery, developed
a spinal metastasis of her prolactinoma which was characterized by rising PRL-levels despite increasing dosages of DA-
agonists. This spinal metastasis turned out to be almost
completely unresponsive to DA-agonist therapy (Fig. 2.). Two
further patients with documented prolactinoma metastases in
the central nervous system have been reported (22,23).

OPERATIVE TREATMENT AND RADIOTHERAPY

Though in patients with microadenomas transsphenoidal
surgery results in normalization of PRL-levels in the majority
of patients, very few subjects with large prolactinomas have
normal prolactin levels after operation (1,5). In addition,

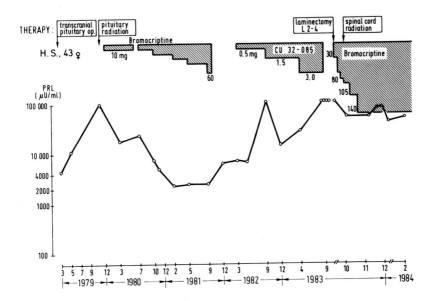

Fig. 2. Spinal metastasis of a pituitary prolactinoma after surgery and radiotherapy. Despite high dosages of bromocriptine PRL-levels remain elevated indicating loss of dopamine receptors by the spinal tumor. The latter shown to be a prolactinoma by immunohistochemistry. There was no adenoma recurrence detectable at cranial CT.

in patients with normalized PRL-levels after transsphenoidal surgery, recurrences in up to 50% of the patients may occur (24).

Radiotherapy with 4500 rad has been applied to patients with hyperprolactinemia. However, the efficacy of this treatment in lowering PRL-levels is poorly documented an varies in individual patients (1,5). Complete normalization of PRL-secretion after radiotherapy in patients with macroprolactinomas is rarely observed (1). Therefore this therapy should be reserved for those patients who are inoperable and do not respond to DA-agonist treatment.

TABLE 1

Clinical appearance of prolactinomas

Parameter	Small adenoma ("microadenoma")	Large invasive macroadenoma
Sex distribution	mainly females	females/males
Proliferation rate	slow	rapid
Elevation of pro-lactin level	moderate	excessive
Visual field de-fects	none	frequent
Neurosurgery	mostly successful	no PRL-normalization
DA-agonist ther-apy (normalization of PRL-levels)	effective	effective
DA-agonist ther-apy (adenoma shrinkage)	?	50 - 80%
Persistent sup-pression after ces-sation of DA-agonist therapy	none	frequent

PREGNANCY IN PROLACTINOMA PATIENTS

Pregnancy is an important therapeutic goal in the hyper-prolactinemic female which can be achieved in the majority of the cases after DA-agonist treatment (5,25). Those females who do not show normalization of PRL-levels during DA-agonist therapy can be treated with pulsatile GnRH-administration. The latter has been shown to enable uneventful pregnancies in persistently hyperprolactinemic patients (26). However, women with prolactinomas may develop complications during preg-nancy. Haemorrhagic phenomena inside the adenoma may lead to sudden increase in tumor size, leading to blindness, cranial nerve palsy or fatal intracranial haemorrhage (for review see 1).

Magyar and Marshall (27) reported about 91 pregnancies occurring in 73 women harbouring an untreated pituitary adenoma. In 23% visual field disturbances and in 25% headaches were reported. In 14 patients symptoms were severe enough to necessitate surgical treatment during pregnancy. Of all 73 patients who became pregnant without prior therapy for the pituitary adenoma, 69 had no permanent *sequelae* after pregnancy. Only 4 patients who were operated on and received radiotherapy developed permanent mild visual field defects. In contrast, 78 pregnancies were observed in 73 females whose prolactinomas had been treated previously. In these patients only 4% developed headaches and 5% visual field disturbances, only one patient requiring treatment during pregnancy.

Gemzell and Wang (28) reviewing the outcome of 217 pregnancies in 187 patients with pituitary adenomas observed uneventful pregnancies in almost all patients with microprolactinomas whereas one quarter of the patients with untreated macroprolactinomas had complications during pregnancy related to the pituitary tumor.

Griffith *et al.* (29) reported on 137 patients harbouring prolactinomas. Of the 116 completed pregnancies, 8 were accompanied by visual field disturbances and 9 by severe headaches.

Rjosk *et al.* (25) reported the outcome of 82 pregnancies in 62 patients with hyperprolactinemic anovulation. Thirty-four pregnancies occurred in patients with a normal *sella turcica* and 25 in women with an intrasellar prolactinoma. Though all subjects were treated with bromocriptine alone, no complications related to the *sella turcica* were observed. Thus, patients with adenomas and no evidence of suprasellar extension before pregnancy have no related morbidity during gestation if hyperprolactinemic sterility had been treated with DA-agonists or GnRH alone. The PRL-levels during pregnancy may differ widely in individual patients (25). Although a steep increase in PRL-levels during pregnancy signals enhanced oestrogen sensitivity, the fact that PRL-levels 3 months after pregnancy can be within the same range as before and excludes growth of the adenoma (25).

In contrast, resolution of hyperprolactinemia after pregnancy can be observed. In 6 out of 62 patients a sudden decrease in the PRL-levels was noted after an initial elevation following bromocriptine withdrawal in the first trimester of pregnancy (25). Resumption of ovulatory cycles after delivery in these patients documented that the anterior pituitary lobe had not been affected and hyperprolactinemia had subsided by spontaneous reduction of the tumor mass.

TABLE 2

Therapy of prolactinomas

Treatment	normal sella	microadenoma or small adenoma	large (invasive) adenoma
Medical therapy	+++	+++	+++
Transsphenoidal surgery	Ø	++	+++ (before pregnancy);++ (after medical therapy)
Radiotherapy	Ø	Ø	(no response to DA-therapy)
Observation only	++ (no clinical symptoms)	++ (no clinical symptoms)	Ø

In patients with macroprolactinomas extending into the sphenoid *sinus* and into the suprasellar area surgery before pregnancy is sometimes necessary in order to prevent gestational complications (1,5,25). Since operative results are less satisfiying in larger adenomas, persisting hyperprolactinemia has to be treated subsequently with DA-agonists. Occasionally, large doses of bromocriptine have to be given over a long period of time to normalize high postoperative PRL-levels (1,15). However, also in these patients radical neurosurgical intervention is not advisable since gonadotrophic function may deteriorate despite normalization of prolactin levels.

REFERENCES

1. Flückiger, F., del Pozo, E. and von Werder, K. (1982). *In* "Monographs in Endocrinology", Vol. 23, Springer, Berlin, Heidelberg, New York.
2. Jung, R.T., White, M.C., Bowley, N.B., Bydder, G., Mashiter, K. and Joplin, G.F. (1982). *Brit. Med. J.* 285, 1078-1081.
3. Editorial (1980). *Lancet* 2, 517-519.
4. Robert, F. (1983). *In* "Prolactin and Prolactinomas" (Eds G. Tolis, C. Stefanis, T. Mountokalakis and F. Labrie). pp. 339-349. Raven Press,New York.

5. von Werder, K., Eversmann, T., Fahlbusch, R. and Rjosk,
    H.K. (1982). *In* "Frontiers in Neuroendocrinology"
    (Eds W.F. Ganong and L. Martini). pp. 123-159. Raven
    Press, New York.
6. Connell, J.M.C., Padfield, P.L., Bunting, E.A., Ball,
    S.G., Inglis, G.C., Bestall, G.H., Teasdale, G.M. and
    Davies, D.L. (1983). *Clin. Endocrinol.* **18**, 527-532.
7. Völker, W., Gehring, W.G., Berning, R., Schmidt, R.C.,
    Schneider, J. and v.z. Mühlen, A. (1982). *Acta Endocr.*
    101, 491-500.
8. Chiodini, P.G., Liuzzi, A., Cozzi, R., Verde, G., Oppizzi,
    G., Dallabonzana, D., Spelta, B., Silvestrini, F.,
    Borghi, G., Luccarelli, G., Rainer, E. and Horowski,
    R. (1981). *J. Clin. Endocr.* **53**, 737-743.
9. Wass, J.A.H., Williams, J., Charlesworth, M., Kingsley,
    D.P.E., Halliday, A.M., Doniach, I., Rees, L.H.,
    McDonald, W.I., Besser, G.M. (1982). *Brit. Med. J.*
    284, 1908-1911.
10. Wollesen, F., Andersen, T. and Karle, A. (1982). *Ann.
    Intern. Med.* **96**, 281-286.
11. del Pozo, E., Gerber, L. and Hunziker, S. (1983). *In*
    "Prolactin and Prolactinomas" (Eds G. Tolis, C.
    Stefanis, T. Mountokalakis and F. Labrie). pp. 403-
    414, Raven Press, New York.
12. Thorner, M.O., Perryman, R.L., Rogol, A.D., Conway, B.P.,
    Mac Leod, R.M., Login, I.S. and Morris, J.L. (1981).
    J. Clin. Endocrinol. **53**, 480-483.
13. Tindall, G.T., Kovacs, K., Horvath, E. and Thorner, M.O.
    (1982). *J. Clin. Endocrinol. Metab.* **55**, 1178-1183.
14. Basetti, M., Spada, A., Pezzo, G. and Giannatasio, G.
    (1984). *J. Clin. Endocr. Metab.* **58**, 268-273.
15. Nissim, M., Ambrosi, B., Bernasconi, V., Giannatasio, G.,
    Giovanelli, M.A., Bassetti, M., Vaccari, U., Moriondo,
    P., Spada, A., Travaglini, P. and Faglia, G. (1982).
    J. Endocrinol. Invest. **5**, 409-415.
16. Eversmann, T., Fahlbusch, R., Rjosk, H.K. and von Werder,
    K. (1979). *Acta Endocrinol.* **92**, 413-427.
17. Winkelmann, W., Allolio, B., Heesen, D., Kaulen, D.,
    Keymer, E. and Mies, R. (1983). *Acta Endocrinol.* (Kbh)
    102, Suppl. **253**, 37-38.
18. von Werder, K. (1984). *In* "Proceedings of the 3rd Europ.
    Workshop on Pituitary Adenomas, Amsterdam, 1983"
    (in press).
19. Landolt, A.M., Keller, P.J., Frösch, E.R. and Müller, J.
    (1982). *Lancet* II, 657-658.
20. Faglia, G., Moriondo, P., Travaglini, P. and Giovanelli,
    M.A. (1983). *Lancet* I, 133-134.

21. Dallabonzana, D., Spelta, B., Oppizzi, G., Tonon, C., Luccarelli, G., Chiodini, P.G. and Liuzzi, A. (1983). *J. Endocrinol. Invest.* 6, 47-50.
22. Martin, N.A., Males, M. and Wilson, C.B. (1981). *J.* Neurosurg.55, 615-619.
23. Cohen, D.L., Dienghdoh, J.V., Thomas, D.G.T. and Himsworth, R.L. (1983). *Clin. Endocrinol.* 18, 259-264.
24. Serri, O., Rasio, E., Beauregard, H., Hardy, J. and Sommer, M. (1983). *N. Engl. J. Med.* 309, 280-283.
25. Rjosk, H.K., Fahlbusch, R. and von Werder, K. (1982). *Acta Endocrinol.* 100, 337-346.
26. Berg, D., Rjosk, H.K., Jänicke, F. and von Werder, K. (1983). *Geburtsh. und Frauenheilk.* 43, 686-688.
27. Magyar, D.M. and Marshall, J.R. (1978). *Am. J. Obstet. Gynaecol.* 132, 739-751.
28. Gemzell, C. and Wang, C.F. (1979). *Fertil. Steril.* 31, 363-372.
29. Griffith, R.W., Turkalj, I. and Braun, P. (1979). *Br. J. Clin. Pharmac.* 7, 393-396.

NEW DEVELOPMENTS IN THE TREATMENT OF HYPERPROLACTINEMIA

S.W.J. Lamberts

Department of Medicine
Erasmus University, Rotterdam, the Netherlands

Dopamine agonists can be considered today as the standard
therapy for patients with PRL-secreting pituitary tumors.
Especially because of the high incidence of recurrences of
hyperprolactinemia after initially successful selective
transsphenoidal operation in patients with microprolactinomas (1), there seems to be no other therapy that can match
the effectiveness of dopamine agonists to normalize PRL levels (in over 95%), to restore fertility and potency (in 80%
to 90%) and to induce considerable shrinkage of the tumors
(in over 75% of the cases;2-4). In this chapter two new aspects of the treatment of hyperprolactinemia will be discussed:

(a) The place and mechanism of action of mesulergine (CU
32-085) in the treatment of hyperprolactinemia.

(b) The treatment of patients with hyperprolactinemia who
showed a low sensitivity to dopamine agonists with antiestrogenic drugs.

RESULTS

(a) *Mesulergine (CU 32-085)*

Bromocriptine, a semi-synthetic ergot alkaloid with a
strong PRL-release-inhibitory effect of comparatively long
duration, inhibits physiologically and pathologically elevated plasma PRL concentrations in man (2,3). It is generally
accepted that its action at least in patients with pituitary
tumors is mediated via a direct inhibitory effect on dopamine receptors on the PRL-secreting tumor cells. This concept is underlined by the data shown in Fig. 1, in which 500
nM dopamine and bromocriptine directly inhibit PRL release
by cultured human pituitary tumor cells, while the dopamine

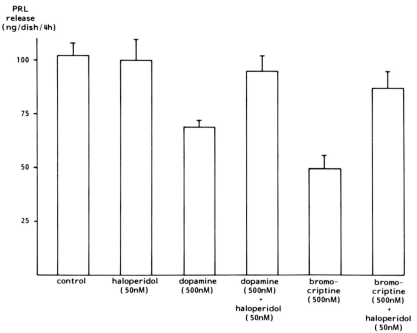

Fig. 1. The effect of dopamine, bromocriptine and haloperidol on the PRL release by cultured tumor cells from a 62-yr-old male patient with a PRL-secreting pituitary macroadenoma. The experiment was carried out for 4 h on day 4 of culture.

receptor antagonist haloperidol (50 nM) completely overcomes these effects.Several classes of drugs have been developed which inhibit PRL secretion (3,5). The ergolines are the most successful ones with a variety of compounds of clinical interest(bromocriptine, lisuride, pergolide and most recently mesulergine: CU 32-085).Peripheral serotonin antagonists like methysergide and metergoline have also been shown to inhibit PRL secretion directly or after metabolization by activation of pituitary dopamine receptors (6,7).

The incidence of adverse effects at the start of treatment with most dopamine agonists is quite high: nausea,vomiting and orthostatic blood pressure changes frequently occur (2). The occurrence of adverse reactions decreases by taking the drugs with meals,but even during chronic treatment with low doses of bromocriptine(up to 10 mg/day) discontinuation of the drug because of side effects took place in 6% of the patients with galactorrhea-amenorrhea.

Recently, mesulergine (CU 32-085) was synthesized. This 8 α-amino-ergoline exerted strong dopaminergic effects in

animals without important actions on the circulation, while
it was less emetic than other comparable drugs (8). The PRL-
lowering effect of mesulergine is about 5 times more potent
than that of bromocriptine. This is shown in Fig. 2,in which
the effects of 0.5 mg mesulergine and 2.5 mg bromocriptine
were compared on plasma PRL levels of a patient with a PRL-
secreting macroadenoma. The acute suppressing effect of the
two compounds was similar but mesulergine exerted a more
prolonged PRL-release-inhibiting effect as plasma PRL levels
remained about 20% of baseline values after 24 h. An important aspect of mesulergine, however, was the low incidence
of side effects after acute and chronic administration. The

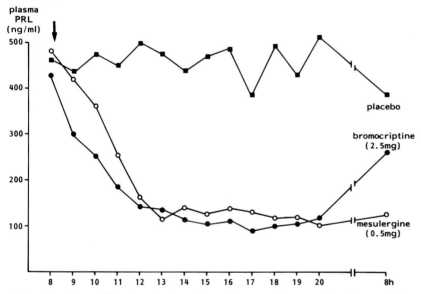

*Fig. 2. The effect of placebo, 2.5 mg bromocriptine and 0.5
mg mesulergine on plasma PRL levels of a 32-yr-old male patient with a PRL-secreting pituitary macroadenoma.*

clinical effects of mesulergine treatment for 16 months were
followed in 6 patients with PRL-secreting pituitary adenomas
who did not tolerate bromocriptine because of persisting
serious side effects of vomiting and hypotension.
    The first dose of mesulergine (0.5 mg) at 08.00 h was
well tolerated without the well-known side effects of other
dopamine agonists. Apart from transient nasal stuffiness
and some dizziness, which disappeared after the second dose
of the drug, no other side effects occurred during treatment
of these patients with 1-2 mg mesulergine per day for 16
months. The PRL-lowering effect of mesulergine and the clin-

ical effects (disappearance of galactorrhea, return of menstrual cycles and fertility and tumor shrinkage)were similar
to those observed in this type of patients during treatment
with bromocriptine.

In order to further investigate the mechanism of action
of mesulergine, experiments were carried out with cultured
normal rat anterior pituitary cells and with the cultured
human tumor cells. In Fig. 3(left) it is shown that 10 nM

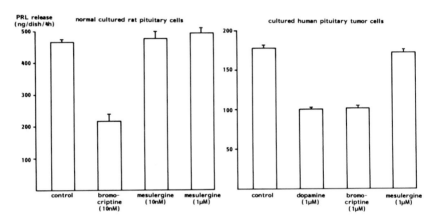

*Fig. 3. The effect of dopamine,bromocriptine and mesulergine
on PRL release by cultured normal rat pituitary cells (left)
and cultured human pituitary tumor cells (right).*

and 1 uM mesulergine were completely ineffective on PRL release by normal rat pituitary cells which were highly sensitive to bromocriptine. This observation was confirmed in a
study with cultured human prolactinoma cells (Fig. 3,right).
Interestingly, it became evident that mesulergine can antagonize the dopamine-mediated inhibition of PRL release by
cultured normal rat pituitary cells in a dose-dependent way
(table 1). Other studies support the observation that mesulergine itself has weak dopamine-receptor antagonistic effects, while one or more metabolites exert the dopaminergic
effects. After parenteral administration, mesulergine was
found to first increase dopamine turnover and DOPAC levels
in the rat striatum, which is followed by a decrease in both
parameters in a time-dependent way(8,9). The lower incidence
of side effects during the use of mesulergine is probably
caused by the anti-dopaminergic action of the compound or by
the slow appearance of the dopamine-agonistic metabolite(s)
after demethylation of the mother compound.

In conclusion, mesulergine is a new PRL-release-inhibiting drug which is well tolerated, even by patients who dis-

continued bromocriptine therapy because of severe nausea,vo-
miting and/or hypotension. The drug is 5 times more potent
and also longer-acting than bromocriptine.Because of the
good tolerance, it might score high in the treatment of ame-
norrhea-galactorrhea, acromegaly and Parkinson's disease.

TABLE 1

*The effect of mesulergine on dopamine-mediated inhibition of
PRL release by normal cultured female rat anterior pituitary
cells*

	PRL release (ng/dish/4h)
control	2033 ± 45
dopamine (DA; 500 nM)	606 ± 13^a
DA (500 nM) + mesulergine (10 nM)	696 ± 28
DA (500 nM) + mesulergine (100 nM)	759 ± 24^b
DA (500 nM) + mesulergine (1 uM)	1473 ± 81^b

Day 4 of culture;incubations for 4 h;mean $\pm$ S.E.M. (n=4)
^{a}p <0.01 vs control ^{b}p <0.01 vs dopamine alone.

(b) *Anti-estrogens*

    The role of estrogens in the regulation of normal PRL se-
secretion in man is uncertain. In the rat it has been made
clear that estrogens stimulate PRL secretion via a stimulating action at three levels (for reviews see 10,11):1)direct
stimulation of PRL release by estrogens at the pituitary level, 2) reduction of dopamine release from the hypothalamus
into the portal vessels reaching the pituitary gland and 3)
impairment of the response of the lactotropic cell to the
inhibitory effect of dopamine. In primates, including man,
in vitro experiments investigating these suggested mechanisms of action of estrogens on PRL secretion at the hypothalamo-pituitary level have not been carried out. In vivo
experiments, however, point to a different effect of estrogens on dopamine-mediated inhibition of PRL release: both in
stalk-sectioned monkeys and in hypogonadal women the effect
of dopamine was shown to be considerably amplified by pretreatment with estrogens (12,13).
    Pharmacological doses of estrogens stimulate both normal
and pathological PRL release, while PRL-secreting pituitary
tumors in man may enlarge during pregnancy as a result of
the increased concentrations of circulating estrogens (3).
Little is known, however, about the effect of estrogens on
the sensitivity of PRL secretion to dopamine or bromocriptine in prolactinoma patients.Chronic administration of the

estrogen receptor blocking agent tamoxifen inhibits hormone
release and the growth of transplantable PRL-secreting pitui
tary tumors in the rat (14,15) and the addition of tamoxifen
to dispersed pituitary tumor cells prepared from these rat
tumors considerably enhances their sensitivity to the inhibitory effects of dopamine and bromocriptine (16).

In 10 patients with invasive PRL-secreting pituitary adenomas with extrasellar extension, we investigated the effect
of tamoxifen on plasma PRL levels and on the bromocriptine-
mediated inhibition of PRL release.Treatment for 5 days with
tamoxifen (20 mg/day) suppressed plasma PRL concentrations
(5 samples measured over the day) significantly in 5 patients by 31+4% (mean $\pm$ SEM;p <0.01 in each individual),while
this decrease was also significant in the group as a whole
(-22+4%;p <0.01). During tamoxifen administration, the inhibitory effect of 2.5 mg bromocriptine (as measured in 10
plasma samples taken hourly from 3 till 12h after this dose)
was also significantly greater in 6 out of these 10 patients
by 47+6% (p <0.05 or p< 0.01 in each individual),while this
increased sensitivity to bromocriptine was also significant
during the use of tamoxifen in the group as a whole (plasma
PRL levels 33+7% lower than after bromocriptine alone; p <
0.01). More details about this study in part of these patients have been published earlier (17).

TABLE 2

The effect of estradiol (10 nM) for 4 days and the acute ad-
ministration of tamoxifen (100 nM) on the sensitivity of
cultured human prolactinoma cells to bromocriptine (10 nM)

	PRL release (ng/dish/4h)	
	control medium (MEM + 10% FCS)	+ estradiol (MEM + 10% FCS + 10 nM E_2)
Patient A		
control	40.0 ± 5.2	73.8 ± 5.8[c]
tamoxifen (100 nM)	38.1 ± 3.8[b]	72.1 ± 4.7
bromocriptine (10 nM)	22.4 ± 3.3[b]	65.2 ± 5.2[b]
tamoxifen+bromocriptine	23.9 ± 6.1[a]	34.9 ± 3.7[b]
Patient B		
control	26.4 ± 2.9	27.6 ± 3.1
tamoxifen (100 nM)	24.9 ± 1.3[b]	29.5 ± 2.5
bromocriptine (10 nM)	18.2 ± 1.2[b]	29.4 ± 2.0[b]
tamoxifen+bromocriptine	19.1 ± 2.3[a]	19.8 ± 2.1[b]

Incubation time 4 h; mean $\pm$ SEM (n = 4)
[a]p< 0.05 vs control   [b]p< 0.01 vs control   [c]p <0.01 vs control without E_2

In vitro experiments with cultured human pituitary tumor cells are in agreement with these observations (table 2A)and suggest a direct interrelation between estrogens, anti-estro gens and dopamine (agonists) at the level of the pituitary tumor. PRL release by the cultured tumor cells of patient 1 was significantly suppressed by bromocriptine (10 nM),while tamoxifen (100 nM) did not affect basal, nor the bromocrip-tine-mediated inhibition of PRL release. Exposure of the cells for 4 days to 10 nM estradiol significantly stimulated PRL release, while the sensitivity to bromocriptine vanished. Tamoxifen itself did not acutely exert an effect,but it made the tumor cells highly sensitive to bromocriptine again.Si-milar results were observed in the tumor cells from another patient (table 2B). In this case, however, estradiol did not stimulate PRL release, but bromocriptine sensitivity was a-gain restored by tamoxifen.

We showed that tamoxifen administration in vivo results in a small but significant suppression of PRL release in part of the patients with giant invasive prolactinomas,while it exerts an additive or potentiating effect on bromocrip-tine-mediated inhibition of PRL secretion in the presence of estrogens. A similar observation was recently reported in 6 of 10 patients in another study (18). The in vitro studies using human pituitary tumor cells support the concept that in pathological circumstances the same estrogen-induced im-pairment of the sensitivity of PRL release to dopamine(ago-nists) is present, as it has also been observed in some rat pituitary tumors in rodents (16). In at least part of the prolactinoma patients anti-estrogens seem to facilitate the inhibitory effect of bromocriptine on PRL secretion. This could mean that chronic treatment of patients with giant prolactinomas with tamoxifen and bromocriptine might result especially in those who show a low sensitivity to bromocrip-tine in a more pronounced reduction in tumor size than bro-mocriptine treatment alone. A definitive conclusion regar-ding the value of tamoxifen treatment in this type of pat-ients has to wait, however, for the results of a double-blind study in which dopamine agonists alone or in combina-tion with tamoxifen are given for a longer period.

REFERENCES

1.   Serri, O., Rasio, E., Beauregard, H., Hardy, J. and
        Somma, M. (1983). *New Engl. J. Med.* 309, 280-283.
2.   Thorner, M.O., Flückiger, E. and Calne, B.D.(1980). *In*
        "Bromocriptine. A Clinical and Pharmacological Review".
        pp. 1-181. Raven Press, New York.

3. Flückiger, E., del Pozo, E. and von Werder, K. (1982).
    In "Prolactin. Physiology, Pharmacology & Clinical
    Findings". pp. 1-224. Springer-Verlag, Berlin.
4. Robinson, A.G. and Nelson, P.B. (1983). *Ann. Int. Med.*
    <u>99</u>, 115-118.
5. Flückiger, E., Vigouret, J.M. and Wagner, H.R. (1978).
    In "Progress in Prolactin Physiology and Pathology"
    (Eds C. Robyn and M. Harter). pp. 383-396. Elsevier/
    North Holland Biomedical Press, Amsterdam.
6. Lamberts, S.W.J. and MacLeod, R.M. (1978). *Endocrinology*
    <u>103</u>, 287-295.
7. Lamberts, S.W.J. and MacLeod, R.M. (1979a). *Proc. Soc.*
    Exp. Biol. Med. <u>162</u>, 75-79.
8. Flückiger, E., Briner, U., Bürki, H.R., Marbach, P.,
    Wagner, H.R. and Doepfner, W. (1979). *Experientia*
    <u>35</u>, 1677-1678.
9. Enz,A. (1981). *Life Sci.* <u>29</u>, 2227-2234.
10. Neill, J.D. (1974). *In* "Handbook of Physiology, Section
    7, Endocrinology vol. IV: The Pituitary Gland and its
    Neuroendocrine Control, part 2" (Eds E. Knobil and
    W.H. Sawyer). pp. 469-488. American Physiological
    Society, Washington, D.C.
11. Franks, S. (1983). *Clin. Sci.* <u>65</u>, 457-462.
12. Neill, J.D., Frawley, L.S., Plotsky, P.M. and Tindall,
    G.T. (1981). *Endocrinology* <u>108</u>, 489-494.
13. Judd, S.J., Rakoff, J.S. and Yen, S.S.C. (1978). *J. Clin.*
    Endocrinol. Metab. <u>47</u>, 494-498.
14. de Quijada, M., Timmermans, H.A.T. and Lamberts, S.W.J.
    (1980). *J. Endocr.* <u>86</u>, 109-116.
15. Nagy, I., Valdenegro, C.A. and MacLeod, R.M. (1980).
    Neuroendocrinology <u>30</u>, 389-395.
16. de Quijada, M., Timmermans, H.A.T., Lamberts, S.W.J. and
    MacLeod, R.M. (1980). *Endocrinology* <u>106</u>, 702-706.
17. Lamberts, S.W.J., Verleun, T. and Oosterom, R. (1982).
    Neuroendocrinology <u>34</u>, 339-342.
18. Völker, W., Gehring, W.G., Berning, R., Schmidt, R.C.,
    Schneider and von zur Mühlen, A. (1982). *Acta Endo-*
    crinol. <u>101</u>, 491-500.

AGE-DEPENDENT EFFECTS OF DOPAMINOMIMETIC
ERGOT COMPOUNDS ON SEX STEROID HORMONES IN RATS

B.P. Richardson and P. Donatsch

*Preclinical Research Department, SANDOZ LTD.,
CH-4002 Basel, Switzerland*

INTRODUCTION

Bromocriptine has established itself as the first of a
new therapeutic class - the directly acting dopaminomimetics. Most, but not all, of its pharmacological and clinical
effects are direct consequences of its ability to stimulate
D_2 receptors (1). It is through a stimulation of such receptors on lactotrophs in the anterior pituitary that bromocriptine reduces prolactin release from these cells, thus
making it a particularly effective drug for the treatment of
a wide variety of clinical conditions associated with increased serum prolactin concentrations (1). Bromocriptine is
also used successfully in the treatment of prolactin-secreting pituitary adenomas, acromegaly and Parkinson's disease.
Although many analogues have been tested in animals and man
subsequently, bromocriptine still remains the best characterized and clinically most useful compound of this type
(2,3).
Although several thousand papers have been published on
the in vivo and in vitro actions of bromocriptine, very few
of these have dealt with the effects of chronic administration in animals. The experiments reported in this communication were prompted by the unexpected finding that treatment
of female rats for one year with bromocriptine produced
squamous metaplasia and hyperplasia of the endometrium which
progressed to pyometritis in some animals. Since these findings were not predictable on the basis of the pharmacological actions of bromocriptine which were known at that time,

DOPAMINE AND NEUROENDOCRINE
ACTIVE SUBSTANCES
ISBN 0 12 209045 4

a series of special experiments were performed to probe the
mechanism by which these effects occur. Ultimately it could
be shown, as described in detail below, that they are not
due to chronic treatment per se, but occur as a result of an
interaction between bromocriptine treatment and the type of
hormonal changes which are characteristic of the waning endocrine system of aging female rats. Thus these effects were
not observed in other species and do not occur in humans.

MATERIALS AND EXPERIMENTAL METHODS

The female rats used for all these studies were OFA Sandoz SPF rats which are a Sprague Dawley-derived strain. This
is an important point because age-related changes in the endocrine system of the female rat, as indicated by vaginal
cytology, vary quite considerably from one strain to the
next. Thus a progression from the regular 4- or 5- day oestrous cycles seen up to the age of about 8 months to irregu-
lar cycles characterized by prolonged oestrous phases
through a subsequent state of constant oestrus, which is
then replaced by a series of pseudopregnancies and ultimately by an anoestrous state at the age of 2-3 years has been
described for one strain of Sprague Dawley rat (4). This also seems to be the case in some strains of Long Evans rats
(5). The OFA Sandoz SPF rats differ from this pattern in
that about 80% of them go from a state of regular oestrous
cycles to pseudopregnancy at the age of 6-8 months without
any intervening period of constant oestrus. They then become
anoestrus at the age of about 16 months. The remaining 20%
show the pattern described above for Long Evans and other
strains of Sprague Dawley rats (6).

Animals were caged singly in an air-conditioned room with
a temperature of $21 \pm 1^{\circ}C$ and relative humidity of $60 \pm 5\%$.
Artificial light was provided from 06.00-18.00 h by fluores-
cent lamps and the animals had free access to a standard
feed (Nafag, Gossau, Switzerland) and water. (Rats were permitted a 10 day acclimatization period before the studies
began.) Vaginal smears were taken each day at 09.00 h and
stained with Giemsa. Bromocriptine and other dopaminomimetic
ergot compounds were given mixed in the feed, except where
otherwise indicated. Progesterone injections were given to
some animals, as indicated in the text and figures, by the
subcutaneous route (1 mg/rat twice daily in 0.1 ml olive
oil). Oestradiol was given in some experiments, twice daily
in olive oil by intramuscular injection. Blood samples which

were drawn at 09.00 h - 11.00 h were obtained by puncture of
the retroorbital venous plexus under light ether narcosis in
most cases. In others, the rats were killed by decapitation
and blood collected from the trunk. Plasma was spun off and
stored at -70°C until estimation of oestradiol and progesterone concentrations by radioimmunoassay was performed. The
mean plasma progesterone and 17β-oestradiol levels of the
different groups were compared statistically using a one-si-
ded analysis of variance and Dunnett's Test (7).

Finally rats were killed by narcosis with CO_2 and exsan-
guination. Ovaries and uteri were dissected out of the animals carefully, inspected and any macroscopic lesions noted.
They were then fixed in Bouin's fixative and prepared for
histology. Haematoxylin and eosin staining was performed
on 5-μm sections.

RESULTS AND DISCUSSION

Effects of Chronic Bromocriptine Treatment on the Rat Ovary and Uterus

The results are shown in Table 1. Treatment with 20
mg/kg/day p.o. bromocriptine for 13 weeks caused an obvious
increase in ovarian size and weight (controls: 0.12 g $\pm$
0.02, treated 0.24 g $\pm$ 0.06; P <0.001), which was due to
the presence of a large number of abnormally formed corpora
lutea. This was not unexpected, since prolactin is known
to be responsible for luteolysis in the rat (8,9). Thus the
reduced prolactin secretion caused by bromocriptine resulted
in an accumulation of non-functional corpora lutea. The
macroscopic and microscopic appearance of the uteri did not
differ from that of age-matched controls.

Treatment at the same dose level for 52 weeks again produced increased numbers of corpora lutea in the ovaries of
the majority, but not all, rats. Five of the 13 treated rats
showed cystic follicles indicative of age-related ovulatory
failure (10). Presumably the increased numbers of corpora
lutea that certainly must have occurred in these rats after
13 weeks treatment had completely regressed during the subsequent months of anovulation, despite the reduced serum
prolactin concentrations. Cystic follicles were also seen
in 4/13 control rats. The uteri of treated rats showed a
picture of oestrogen dominance: squamous metaplasia and hyperplasia of the endometrium, which had progressed to endo-
metritis and pyometritis in many animals. This was totally

unpredictable on the basis of the pharmacological actions
which were known for bromocriptine at that time. This prompted the obvious question "Does bromocriptine possess direct
oestrogenic activity?".

TABLE 1

*Histological findings in the ovaries and uteri of rats
treated with bromocriptine (20 mg/kg/day p.o.)*

ORGAN	13 Weeks Treatment		52 Weeks Treatment	
	Controls	Bromocriptine	Controls	Bromocriptine
OVARIES				
Increased abnormal corpora lutea	0/5	10/10	0/13	7/12
Cystic follicles	1/5	2/10	4/13	5/12
UTERUS				
Endometrial hyper-plasia				
- slight	2/5	4/10	8/13	5/13
- moderate	0/5	0/10	0/13	5/13
Endometrial squamous metaplasia	0/5	0/10	0/13	2/13
Pyometritis/ Endometritis	0/5	0/10	0/13	6/13

Test for Direct Oestrogenic Activity of Bromocriptine in Rats

Groups of 10 adult ovariectomized rats with proven responsiveness to exogenous oestradiol (100 μg/kg induced an oestrus vaginal smear) received either bromocriptine (5, 20 or
80 mg/kg twice orally) or estradiol (0.001, 0.003, 0.01 or
0.03 mg/kg twice intramuscularly). The two administrations
were given 8 hours apart and appropriate controls were run
with vehicles. Vaginal smears were taken at intervals up to
64 hours after the second administration, and then the rats
were killed and the uterine horns dissected out and weighed.

Bromocriptine failed to induce changes in vaginal smear cytology whereas oestradiol produced dose-dependent squamous metaplasia. The relative uterine weights of the oestradiol--treated rats were dose-dependently increased compared with the controls whereas those of the bromocriptine-treated rats were unchanged.

These results show that bromocriptine does not possess direct oestrogenic activity in rats.

The next question that we asked was "Does bromocriptine elevate absolute or relative endogenous oestrogen levels in rats?"

Plasma Oestradiol and Progesterone Levels in Rats Treated Chronically with Bromocriptine

Eight-week old rats were treated orally for 2 years with 10 mg/kg/day bromocriptine. Figure 1 shows that plasma oestradiol levels in control rats were similar at 14 and 60 weeks of age and declined thereafter. This pattern is similar to that reported for other rat strains (11,12). There was no significant difference between the oestradiol levels found in control and bromocriptine-treated rats at any time point when this parameter was measured.

Plasma progesterone concentrations also showed age-related changes. In control rats there was a pronounced increase between 14 and 60 weeks of age. This, as will be shown later, is related to the development of the state of pseudopregnancy, and is a phenomenon which is also reported in the literature for other strains of rat (11, 12,13). After 60 weeks of age the plasma progesterone levels declined, although they were still five times higher than at 14 weeks of age. There was no difference in the plasma progesterone levels of control and bromocriptine-treated rats after 6 weeks' treatment. Thereafter however, bromocriptine totally abolished the age-related increase, the plasma progesterone concentrations of treated rats remaining virtually constant throughout the study (i.e. approximately 5 ng/ml). It will be seen in the studies described below that this occurs because bromocriptine, by virtue of its ability to inhibit prolactin release, prevents pseudopregnancy occurring in treated rats. Hence the progesterone levels of bromocriptine rats were significantly lower than controls at treatment weeks 52 and 78 (i.e. when rats were 60 and 86 weeks old respectively). If one studies the progesterone:oestradiol

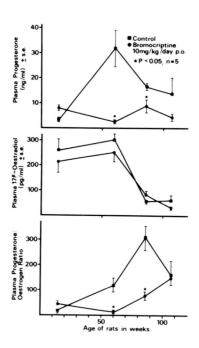

Fig. 1. Plasma progesterone, 17β-oestradiol and progesterone: oestradiol ratio of control and bromocriptine-treated female OFA rats. Treatment with bromocriptine was started when the rats were 8 weeks old. The drug was given mixed in the feed.

ratios in controls with time there is an increase up until 86 weeks of age and then a decline. Bromocriptine treatment caused a very large and statistically significant reduction in this ratio at treatment weeks 52 and 78, that is to say it induced relative hyperoestrogenism for a large part of the study. This progesterone:oestrogen inbalance could certainly explain the pattern of oestrogen dominance observed in the uteri of rats treated with bromocriptine for one year. Therefore the next question that we asked was "Is the relative hyperoestrogenism caused by bromocriptine due to chronic treatment per se, or does it occur as a result of relatively acute effects superimposed on the waning endocrine system of the aging female OFA rats?"

*Effects of Bromocriptine on the Vaginal Smear Pattern of
Young and Old rats*

The detailed results of these studies has already been
reported elsewhere (6). Groups of 10 young (8-11 weeks old)
and 10 old (38-42 weeks old) female rats were used. Only
rats showing regular 4 or 5 day cyclical vaginal smear patterns were selected. Ninety percent of the younger group
displayed these compared with only 40% of the older group.
The remaining 60% of the older groups showed prolonged periods of dioestrus i.e. pseudopregnancy as described for
other rat strains (4,13,14).

After 2 weeks of medication bromocriptine produced markedly different responses in the vaginal smear patterns of
young and old rats (see Table 2A and B). Old control rats
showed prolonged periods of dioestrus with increasing frequency whilst the treated group showed double oestrous
and subsequently persistent vaginal cornification associated
with the presence of developing and cystic follicles in the
ovaries. This phenomenon was dose-dependent. It was not observed in continuously-treated young rats until they
achieved the same age as the older group (i.e. after 12-15
weeks' medication). Thus by preventing pseudopregnancy, bromocriptine increased the incidence of the alternative phase
for old rats i.e. one of persistent vaginal cornification.
Old rats stay in this phase because inadequacies in their LH
surge mechanism prevent the successful ovulation of mature
follicles from the ovary (10,13,15,16). This situation may
have been aggravated by an additional inhibitory effect of
bromocriptine on the preovulatory LH surge at high doses
(17). Such retained follicles can subsequently become cystic.

The presence of cystic follicles and persistent vaginal
cornification led to squamous metaplasia of the uterine endometrium and eventually to pyometra whereas the presence
of excessive numbers of corpora lutea alone (indicative of
prolactin inhibition) had no effect on either the vaginal
smear pattern or on the endometrium. From the foregoing it
can be concluded that cystic follicles, squamous metaplasia
of the endometrium and pyometra are not merely the effects
of long term oral administration of bromocriptine to rats,
since they only result when medication is superimposed upon
a waning endogenous endocrine system. Thus the action of
bromocriptine to prevent pseudopregnancy and induce a state
of constant oestrus in old OFA rats apparently relies simply
on its ability to lower serum prolactin. In keeping with

Table 2

Effects of oral bromocriptine administration on vaginal smear patterns in young and old rats

A. *Number of rats showing dioestrus periods longer than 5 days (10 rats/group)*

Week of Treatment	Young Rats			Old Rats		
	Control	Bromocriptine		Control	Bromocriptine	
		5 mg/kg	83 mg/kg		5 mg/kg	83 mg/kg
1	0	0	0	0	0	0
2	1	0	0	4	0	0
3	1	0	0	5	0	0
5	3	0	0	6	0	0
10	4	0	0	8	0	0
15	6	0	0	8	0	0
20	8	1	0	8	0	0

B. *Number of rats showing persistent vaginal cornification (10 rats/group)*

Week of Treatment	Young Rats			Old Rats		
	Control	Bromocriptine		Control	Bromocriptine	
		5 mg/kg	83 mg/kg		5 mg/kg	83 mg/kg
1	0	0	0	0	0	0
2	0	0	0	0	0	2
3	0	0	0	0	0	4
5	0	0	0	0	2	7
10	0	0	1	1	4	9
15	0	0	3	1	4	9
20	0	0	4	2	5	10

this notion is the fact that a large number of dopaminergic compounds which reduce prolactin secretion produce essentially identical results. These include compounds such as lisuride which have been synthesized by research groups working in other pharmaceutical companies.

The exact mechanism by which the constant oestrous vaginal smear pattern and oestrogen-dominated endometrial changes occurred in bromocriptine was the subject of the experiment described below.

Correlation Between Effects of Bromocriptine on Vaginal Smear Pattern and Plasma Steroid Levels in Old Pseudopregnant Rats

Two groups of 30 old (37-60 weeks old) pseudopregnant rats were used for this study. One group was treated with 10 mg/kg/day bromocriptine, the other acted as control. At various time points groups of 5 treated rats were removed from the study, killed by decapitation and plasma samples collected for progesterone and oestradiol estimation. Vaginal smears were recorded throughout.

The results are summarized in Figure 2. The upper panel shows the vaginal smear pattern of a typical treated rat. Bromocriptine interrupted pseudopregnancy and initiated cyclical vaginal smear patterns in all 30 rats. This was expected, since pseudopregnancy is a condition where active, progesterone-secreting, corpora lutea are maintained in the ovary by inappropriate prolactin secretion, as mentioned previously. Similar effects have been reported with other dopaminergic compounds such as lergotrile and L-DOPA (4,14). Figure 2 shows that inhibiting prolactin secretion with bromocriptine indeed led to a statistically significant lowering of plasma progesterone concentration and consequent reduction in progesterone:oestradiol ratio, and that this was associated with reinitiation of regular cyclical changes in the vaginal smear patterns. In fact it has been suggested that the combination of high serum progesterone and oestradiol which occurs in pseudopregnant rats blocks the surges in pituitary gonadotropin secretion which are necessary for regular cyclical ovarian activity (12). Bromocriptine-treated rats subsequently continued to show regular oestrous cycles for 2-3 weeks. As time progressed, many rats started to display double oestrous days, indicative of ovulatory failure. Soon afterwards all rats showed persistent vaginal cornifi-

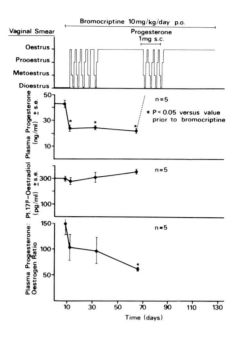

Fig. 2. Effects of bromocriptine treatment on the vaginal smear pattern, plasma progesterone and 17β-oestradiol concentrations and progesterone: oestradiol ratios of old pseudopregnant OFA rats. Bromocriptine was given in the feed. When rats displayed constant oestrus, 1 mg progesterone/rat was given subcutaneously in olive oil twice daily.

cation (constant oestrus) which was associated with a further reduction in plasma progesterone and progesterone:oestradiol ratio. This increasing tendency to anovulation results as a consequence of the well recognized deficiency in the preovulatory LH surge which occurs in senescent rats (4,13,16,18). It is also possible that this may have been accentuated by an additional inhibitory effect of bromocriptine on the LH surge (17). Old rats which display constant oestrus spontaneously can be made to ovulate and show regular cyclical vaginal smear patterns by injections of progesterone (4), presumably because progesterone is a potent stimulus for LH release (16). As can be seen from Figure 2, progesterone was also effective in reinitiating cyclical vaginal smears in bromocriptine-treated rats, suggesting that the aetiology of constant oestrus in old bromocrip-

tine-treated rats is identical to that occurring in some
animals spontaneously. When progesterone injections were
stopped, the cyclical vaginal smear pattern was again replaced by one of constant oestrus within 4 days.

In conclusion it can be said that the state of constant
oestrus which occurs in old OFA rats when treated with dopamine agonists occurs because the usual pseudopregnancy state
is prevented or interrupted. This happens because pseudopregnancy is a prolactin-dependent condition and central
dopamine agonists inhibit pituitary prolactin secretion.
Although old pseudopregnant rats display regular cyclical
vaginal smear patterns after administration of dopamine agonists, this cannot be maintained in the face of a progressive deficiency in the preovulatory LH surge mechanism which
occurs in these old rats. This may be accentuated by an additional LH surge lowering action such prolactin-inhibiting
compounds may have at higher doses. The result is ovulatory
failure and persistent vaginal cornification which occurs
as a manifestation of the low progesterone:oestradiol ratio
seen in these animals. Chronic oestrogen dominance also pro-
duces uterine changes - squamous metaplasia and hyperplasia
of the endometrium which, in some cases, progresses to pyometritis.
From this series of studies it is obvious that the ova-
rio-uterine findings from the one-year rat study are likely
to be species- or even strain-specific and thus irrelevant
for the clinical use of bromocriptine. Thus similar findings
did not occur in a one-year dog study or in a life time
mouse study. More importantly clinical studies have shown
that bromocriptine did not influence FSH, LH, oestradiol
or progesterone levels in 90 hyperprolactinaemic women. As
expected, endometrial biopsies in 88 patients treated with
bromocriptine for 2 to 72 months at doses varying from 1.25
to 60 mg/kg did not show any drug-related changes (19).
The ability to interrupt pseudopregnancy with dopamine
agonists and the subsequent occurrence of ovulation failure
with persistent vaginal cornification are indicative of the
changes in neurotransmitter turnover which occur in the median eminence of these aging rats. It is widely accepted
that the release of prolactin is under the negative control
of a hypothalamic factor that reaches the anterior pituitary
in the portal blood (for review see refs 20,21). Circumstan-
tial evidence seems to suggest that this factor is dopamine
which originates in the tuberoinfundibular dopamine neurones

(20). The fact that serum prolactin is elevated in old rats thus suggests that there may be an age-related decrease in the functioning of this system. This has indeed been recently found (11,22,23). The decrease in functioning appears to be due to a loss of dopamine neurons. The deficit in the tuberoinfundibular system was obviously corrected in our studies by the administration of directly acting dopamine agonists. In this way it was possible to reduce the elevated prolactin secretion and thereby interrupt pseudopregnancy. Since activation of noradrenaline-containing neurones in the hypothalamus may stimulate the release of gonadotropin-releasing factors into the portal blood and hence cause the secretion of LH from the pituitary, the recently reported decrease in noradrenaline content of the hypothalamus may similarly explain the reduced preovulatory LH surge which is found in aging rats (22,23). Consistent with this notion is the fact that injections of adrenaline can initiate regular oestrous cycles in old rats with persistent vaginal cornification (15).

REFERENCES

1. Thorner, M.O., Flückiger, E. and Calne, D.B. (1980). *In* "Bromocriptine. A Clinical and Pharmacological Review". Raven Press, New York.
2. Flückiger, E., Vigouret, J.M. and Wagner, H.R. (1978). *In* "Progress in Prolactin Physiology and Pathology" (Eds C. Robyn and M. Harter), pp. 383-396. Elsevier/ North Holland Biomedical Press, Amsterdam.
3. Flückiger, E. (1980). *In* "Ergot Compounds and Brain Function. Neuroendocrine and Neuropsychiatric Aspects" (Eds M. Goldstein, A. Liebermann, D.B. Calne and M.O. Thorner), pp. 155-163. Raven Press, New York.
4. Meites, J., Huang, H.H. and Riegle, G.D. (1976). *In* "Hypothalamus and Endocrine Functions" (Eds F. Labrie, J. Meites and G. Pelletier), pp. 3-20. Plenum Press, New York and London.
5. Huang, H.H. and Meites, J. (1975). *Neuroendocrinology* 17, 289-295.
6. Flückiger E. *et al.* (1982). *In* "Aging Brain and Ergot Alkaloids" (Eds A. Agnoli, G. Crepaldi, P.F. Spano and M. Trabucchi), pp. 61-71. Raven Press, New York.
7. Dunnett, C.H.W. (1955). *J. Am. Stat. Ass.* 50, 1096-1121.
8. Malven, P.V., Cousar, G.J. and Row, E.H. (1969). *Am. J. Physiol.* 216, 421-424.

9. Billeter, E. and Flückiger, E. (1971). *Experientia* <u>77</u>, 464-465.
10. Clemens, J.A. and Meites, J. (1979). *Neuroendocrinology* <u>7</u>, 249-256.
11. Wilkes, M.M., Lu, K.H., Fulton, S.L. and Yen, S.S.C. (1978). *Adv. exp. Med. Biol.* <u>113</u>, 127-147.
12. Huang, H.H., Steger, R.W., Bruni, J.F. and Meites, J. (1978). *Endocrinology* <u>103</u>, 1855-1859.
13. Wise, P.M. and Ratner, A. (1980). *Neuroendocrinology* <u>30</u>, 15-19.
14. Clemens, J.A. and Fuller, R.W. (1978). *Adv. exp. Med. Biol.* <u>97</u>, 187-206.
15. Clemens, J.A., Amenomori, Y., Jenkins, T. and Meites, J. (1969). *Proc. Soc. exp. Biol. Med.* <u>132</u>, 561-563.
16. Lu, K.H., Huang, H.H., Chen, H.T., Kurcz, M., Mioduszewski, R. and Meites, J. (1977). *Proc. Soc. exp. Biol. Med.* <u>154</u>, 82-85.
17. Markó, M. and Flückiger, E. (1974). *Experientia* <u>30</u>, 1174-1176.
18. McPherson, J.C., Costoff, A. and Makesh, V.B. (1977). *Fertility and Sterility* <u>28</u>, 1365-1370.
19. Besser, G.M., Thorner, M.O., Wass, J.A.H., Doniach, I., Conti, G., Curling, M., Grudziniskas, J.G. and Setchell, M.E. (1977). *Brit. med. J.* <u>II</u>, 868.
20. Lichtensteiger, W. (1979). *In* "The Neurobiology of Dopamine Systems" (Eds A.S. Horn, J. Korf and B.H.C. Westerink), pp. 491-521. Academic Press, London.
21. Flückiger, E., del Pozo, E. and von Werder, K. (1982) *In* "Prolactin. Physiology, Pharmacology and Clinical Findings". Springer Verlag, Berlin.
22. Simpkins, J.W., Mueller, G.P., Huang, H.H. and Meites, J. (1977). *Endocrinology* <u>100</u>, 1672-1678.
23. Demarest, K.T., Riegle, G.D. and Moore, K.E. (1980). *Neuroendocrinology* <u>31</u>, 222-227.

IV. Control of Gonadotropin Release

THE METABOLISM OF TESTOSTERONE IN THE NEUROENDOCRINE STRUCTURES

L. Martini

Department of Endocrinology
University of Milano - 20129 Milano - Italy

INTRODUCTION

A large group of research which may now be labelled as "classical" has demonstrated that the prostate and other androgen-sensitive peripheral structures (seminal vesicles, sebaceous gland, kidney, etc.) metabolize testosterone into 5α-androstane-17β-ol-3-one (dihydrotestosterone, DHT) and subsequently into 5α-androstane-3α,17β-diol (3-diol)(1). In the peripheral androgen-responding tissues small amounts of 5α-androstane-3β-,17β-diol (3β-diol) are also formed from DHT (1). These conversions occur under the influence of an enzymatic complex that includes a 5α-reductase, and two (3α- and 3β-) hydroxysteroid dehydrogenases. According to a theory which is now generally accepted, the 5α-reduced metabolites represent the intracellular mediators for the multiple actions testosterone exerts in its target structures (2).

There is also ample evidence derived from *in vivo* and *in vitro* studies indicating that in adult male mammals, the anterior pituitary and several central nervous structures (hypothalamus, midbrain, amygdala, etc.) are able to convert testosterone into DHT and 3α-diol (3) (Fig. 1). Actually, the anterior pituitary metabolizes testosterone into DHT and 3α-diol with yields that are second only those found in the prostate and seminal vesicles.

The data are consistent for a large group of species (rat, mouse, dog, monkey, cow and guinea pig)(3). The presence of a 5α-reductase-3α-hydroxysteroid dehydrogenase complex has also been described in the human anterior pituitary and in the human brain (4). The 5α-reducing processes occurring in the brain and anterior pituitary are similar to those described for the peripheral androgen-dependent structures. The only sig-

DOPAMINE AND NEUROENDOCRINE
ACTIVE SUBSTANCES
ISBN 0 12 209045 4

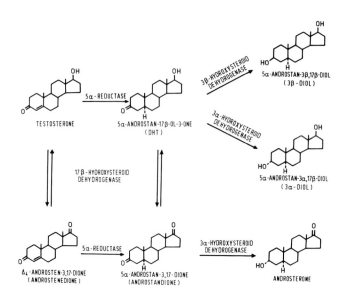

*Fig. 1. Conversion of testosterone into its 5α-reduced metab-
olites by different tissues.*

nificant difference seems to reside in the fact that, in the
central structures, higher amounts of 3α-diol are formed (5).
Similarly to what occurs in the peripheral androgen-responding
structures, minute amounts of 3α-diol are also formed from
DHT in the anterior pituitary and brain.

In the latter, but probably not in the anterior pituitary
of adult animals the 5α-reductase pathway coexists with another
important metabolic system, which, through the process of aromatization, transforms androgens into estrogens (respectively testosterone into estradiol and Δ₄-androstenedione into
estrone)(Fig. 2)(7). In adult animals, the hypothalamus has
been shown to be the most potent aromatizing area, followed
by the limbic system. Although the yields of the aromatization
process are much lower than those provided by the 5α-reductase
system, aromatization may represent an important step in the
expression of some effects of androgens, since, on a molecular
weight basis, estrogens are significantly more potent than
androgens. The perinatal "organization" of the brain towards
male patterns of control of gonadotropin secretion and of sexual behaviour has been ascribed to this aromatization process.
Also, the control of adult male sexual behaviour seems to need
the aromatization of androgens in the CNS (7).

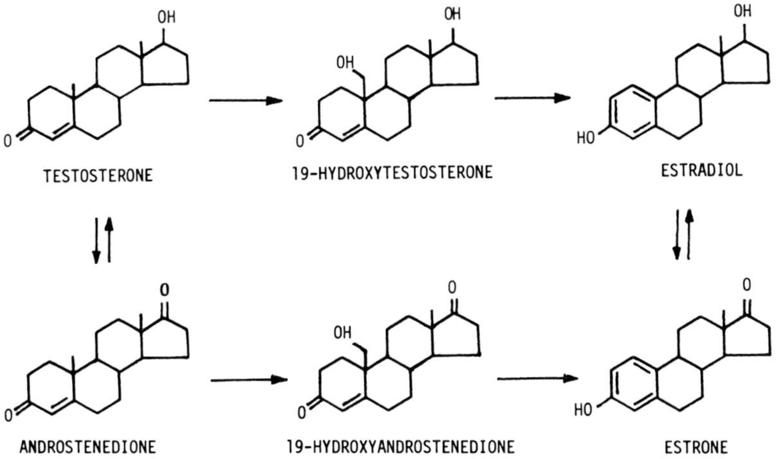

Fig. 2. The aromatase pathway.

It is still a matter of discussion whether, in mammals, the 5α-reductase-3-hydroxysteroid dehydrogenase system is present in all pituitary cells or whether these enzymatic activities are confined only to one cell subpopulation. However, some evidence seems to suggest that 5α-reductase is predominantly (if not exclusively) localized in the gonadotrophs.

Sar and Stumpf (8) have reported that exogenous labelled testosterone is concentrated only in the gonadotrophs. After a sedimentation of monodispersed pituitary cells obtained from normal male rats and their incubation with labelled testoster-One, Lloyd and Karavolas (9) and Denef (10) found that the fraction containing the gonadotrophs forms more DHT than those containing the chromophobes or the somatotropic cells. The preferential localization of 5α-reductase in the gonadotrophs has been substantiated also in an *in vivo* study performed by Celotti *et al.*(11). It is known that, when pituitary tissue is transplanted underneath the kidney capsule of hypophysectomized animals, the gonadotrophs will atrophy and gradually disappear, and that the graft will be mainly formed by prolactin-secreting cells. It is also known that the administration of exogenous LHRH will prevent the disappearance of the gonadotrophs from the grafted pituitary (12). Celotti *et al.* (11) have measured *in vitro* the 5α-reductase activity of pituitary that had been

previously grafted underneath the kidney capsule of hypophysectomized rats. The study included two groups of experimental
animals: one treated with saline and the other with LHRH.
Three days after grafting, a sharp decline in the 5α-reductase
activity was observed in both groups of pituitaries. The enzymatic activity remained low for up to 14 days in the animals
treated with saline; on the contrary, a progressive increase
in the 5α-reductase activity was observed in the animals receiving LHRH substitution therapy.

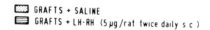

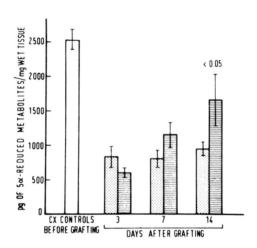

*Fig. 3. In vitro metabolism of testosterone in anterior pitu-
itary homografts from castrated rats placed underneath the
kidney capsule of hypophysectomized rats.*

On the 14th day, the activity of the pituitary graft of the
animals treated with the hypothalamic hormone was significantly higher than that of the corresponding control glands
(Fig. 3). The increase in 5α-reductase activity in the graft
following the administration of LHRH correlated well with the
reappearance of gonadotrophs, as evaluated at the light and
electron microscope level. Indirect support of the thesis that
5α-reductase is predominantly present in the gonadotrophs may
also be derived from those studies which indicate that the
5α-reductase activity of the anterior pituitary is greatly
increased following castration and normalized by the administration of exogenous sex steroids.
    It is known that the gonadotrophs increase in size and
proliferate after orchidectomy and that treatment with either

testosterone or estrogens restores normal pituitary histology
in castrated animals (3),

FACTORS CONTROLLING THE 5α-REDUCTASE OF THE ANTERIOR
PITUITARY AND HYPOTHALAMUS

As previously mentioned it is possible that the increase
in the 5α-reducing ability of the anterior pituitary after
castration reflects the changes in the composition of pituitary cell population that follow the operation, since the gonadotrophs increase in size and proliferate after gonadectomy.
The fact that the 5α-reductase activity of the anterior
pituitary depends on circulating androgens is further substantiated by the observation that, in orchidectomized animals,
the administration of testosterone or of other androgens (DHT,
3α-diol, etc.) restores the enzymatic activity of the gland
to precastration levels (13,14). Estrogens are also able to
decrease the 5α-reductase activity of the anterior pituitary
of castrated male rats. The administration of small doses of
estrogen benzoate for 7 days to castrated rats decreases such
activity to normal levels. It is interesting that continuation
of the treatment for 14 days will induce a further decline
in enzymatic activity in the gland; this will drop to below
the levels found in normal animals (15).
At variance with what occurs at the anterior pituitary level, endogenous androgens seem to exert only minor effects on
the 5α-reductase activity of the hypothalamus of adult male
rats. Castration does not significantly increase the ability
of the hypothalamus to transform testosterone into DHT and
3α-diol (5,13). Conversely, the administration of exogenous
androgens (either in physiological amounts or in dosages
exceeding physiological levels) has been reported by the majority of authors not to decrease the activity of the 5α-reductase
-3α-hydroxysteroid dehydrogenase system of this structure
(5,13,15). The administration of estrogens over a prolonged
period of time (either in physiological or in pharmacological
quantities) is also ineffective in decreasing the 5α-reductase
activity of the hypothalamus of the castrated male rat (15).
This again is at variance with what occurs in the anterior
pituitary.
Environmental light conditions appear to be an important
factor for the control of the 5α-reductase activity of the
hypothalamus. Exposure of adult male rats to constant dark,
but not to constant light, has been reported to decrease the
5α-reductase activity of this structure, without altering that
of the anterior pituitary (16). This finding might suggest that
the pineal gland, a photosensitive structure, intervenes in the

control of the 5α-reductase activity of the hypothalamus.

The possibility that the hypothalamic 5α-reductase might be influenced by neural factors (e.g. brain neurotransmitter) has been recently explored. Only negative results were obtained so far. It has been shown that the administration of drugs such as atrophine, reserpine, p-chlorophenylalanine and naloxone (which respectively alter cholinergic, adrenergic, serotoninergic and opiate-mediated inputs to the hypothalamus) does not alter the testosterone-metabolizing capability of the hypothalamus (17). Also, a total hypothalamic deafferentiation performed according to the classical technique of Halasz remains without effect (17).

ROLE OF TESTOSTERONE METABOLISM IN THE BRAIN AND ANTERIOR PITUITARY

The majority of data available indicate that DHT, when administered systematically (either acutely or chronically), is more effective than testosterone in suppressing LH release. This occurs in all animal species studied so far and in humans (3,18). In the animal species in which it has been tested, systematically administered 3α-diol has been found to be as active as, or more effective than, DHT in inhibiting LH release (3,18)(Fig. 4).

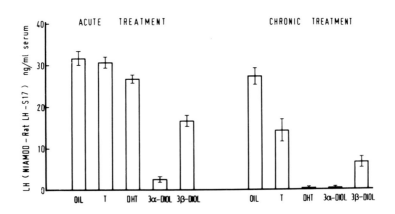

Fig. 4. Effects of treatment with testosterone (T), DHT, 3α-diol and 3β-diol on serum LH levels of adult castrated male rats.

The inhibitory effect of DHT and of 3α-diol is obviously more evident after castration, when serum gonadotropin levels are elevated.

These observations have led to the hypothesis that the formation of DHT and 3α-diol in the neuroendocrine structures might be crucial for the testosterone to exert its negative feedback effect on LH secretion (5,19). An inhibitory effect of 3α-diol on the secretion of this gonadotropin has also been found by some authors but has been denied by others (3,18,19). The effects of this steroid probably depend on the doses, the route of administration and other experimental parameters.

Support for the theory that the process of 5α-reduction is important for the inhibitory control of LH secretion may be derived from an experiment of nature. Recently, a new form of male pseudohermaphroditism has been described in a few kindreds from different geographical locations (Dominican Republic, United States, Cyprus, Algeria, Mexico). In the affected individuals a hereditary deficiency of the 5α-reductase system has been demonstrated. Hence these patients have serum levels of DHT well below normal. In the majority of these hermaphrodites serum LH is elevated despite the presence of normal or high serum levels of testosterone and estrogens (20,21,22,23).

In castrated experimental animals, DHT and 3α-diol are less effective than testosterone in inhibiting the release of FSH (3,18,24,25). Moreover, it has been shown that higher doses of the two steroids are needed to inhibit FSH than to inhibit LH (26). The inefficacy of DHT as a suppressor of FSH secretion has been confirmed also in humans (25), whereas 3α-diol has never been studied in men. These data seem to assign only a secondary role to the 5α-reduced metabolites of testosterone in the negative feedback control of FSH release. Hence it is possible that testosterone intervenes in this control either acting directly or after conversion (in the CNS, in the plasma compartment, in the liver, etc.) to estrogenic molecules (3). These steroids are indeed good suppressors of FSH release.

It is probable that the process of 5α-reduction of testosterone in the brain and anterior pituitary participates in the control of the onset of puberty in male animals. Current theories explain male puberty either as the result of a progressive increase in the sensitivity of the testis to gonadotropins (27), or as the result of a progressive decrease in the sensitivity of the hypothalamic-pituitary axis to the negative feedback effects of androgens (28,29,30,31). According to this theory, lower levels of androgens in the general circulation would be necessary to keep gonadotropin secretion in check in prepuberal than in adult animals, or alternatively,

the same amount of androgens would be more effective in inhibiting gonadotropin secretion before than after puberty
(28,29,30,31). Massa *et al.* (13) have postulated that the
hypersensitivity to androgens of the "gonadostat" in prepubert-
al animals convert testosterone into its "active" LH-inhibit-
ing metabolites (DHT, 3α-diol) more efficiently than those
of adult animals. This hypothesis was verified by analyzing
the 5α-reductase activity of the central structures of male
rats of 1,3,5,7,14,21,28,35 and 60 days of age (32). It was
found that the 5α-reductase activity of the anterior pituitary
was extremely elevated at 1 day of age and showed subsequently
a progressive decline. Also, the 5α-reductase activity of the
hypothalamus was found to be elevated immediately after birth,
to show a further increase between days 1 and 3 of neonatal
life, and to decline subsequently to reach adult levels at
35 days of age (32). The most interesting finding in these

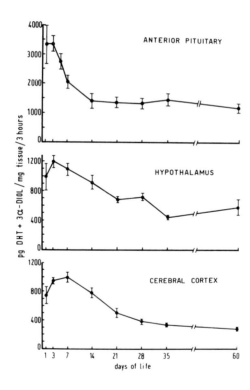

*Fig. 5. In vitro metabolism of testosterone into 5α-reduced
metabolites (DHT + 3α-diol) in different brain structures of
male rats of different ages.*

series of experiments was the observation that also cerebral cortex of neonatal ans young animals possesses significant amounts of 5α-reducing enzymes. In the cerebral cortex, as in the hypothalamus, an increase in this enzymatic activity has been observed during the first days of life. Subsequently a progressive decline was recorded which lasted up to the 35th day (32)(Fig. 5). These findings have been confirmed by Denef *et al.* (33). It is felt that these data might provide a biochemical basis for explaining the changes in the sensivity of the central "gonadostat" that occur at the time of sexual maturation and that seem crucial for the initiation of puberty in male animals. The enhanced formation of DHT and 3α-diol before puberty in the central structures provides the hypothalamic-pituitary complex with steroids that, as previously mentioned, possess an increased capability of inhibiting LH secretion.

ACKNOWLEDGMENTS

The experiments described in the present paper were supported by grants from the Consiglio Nazionale delle Ricerche, Roma, Italy (through the projects "Preventive and Rehabilitative Medicine", "Control of Neoplastic Growth" and "Group of Endocrinology"). Such support is gratefully acknowledged.

REFERENCES

1.   Wilson, J.D. and Gloyna, R.E. (1970). *Recent Progr. Hormone Res.* 26, 309-336.
2.   Schmidt, H., Giba-Tziampiri, O., Rotteck, G. and Voigt, K.D. (1973). *Acta Endocr.* 73, 599-611.
3.   Martini, L. (1982). *Endocrine Rev.* 3, 1-25.
4.   Mickan, H. (1972). *Steroids* 19, 659-666.
5.   Martini, L. (1976). *In* "Subcellular Mechanisms in Reproductive Neuroendocrinology" (Eds F. Naftolin, K.J. Ryan and I.J. Davies), pp. 327-345. Elsevier, Amsterdam.
6.   Genot, A., Loras, B., Monbon, M. and Bertrand, J. (1975). *J. Steroid Biochem.* 6, 1247-1252.
7.   Naftolin, F., Ryan, K.J., Davies, I.J., Reddy, V.V.R., Flores, F., Petro, Z., Kuhn, M., White, R.J., Takaoka, Y. and Wolin, L. (1975). *Recent Progr. Hormone Res.* 31, 295-315.
8.   Sar, M. and Stumpf, W.E. (1973). *Endocrinology* 92, 631-635.
9.   Lloyd, R.V. and Karavolas, H.J. (1975). *Endocrinology* 95, 517-526.

10. Denef, C. (1979). *Neuroendocrinology* 29, 132-139.
11. Celotti, F., Farina, J., Cresti, L., Massa, R. and
    Martini, L. (1976). *In* "Program 5th Intern. Congr.
    Endocrinology", p. 44.
12. McLean, B.K. and Nikitovitch-Winer, M.B. (1976). *Neuro-endocrinology* 20, 1-13.
13. Massa, R., Stupnicka, E., Kniewald, Z. and Martini, L.
    (1972). *J. Steroid Biochem.* 3, 385-399.
14. Celotti, F., Ferraboschi, P., Negri-Cesi, P. and Martini,
    L. (1980). *In* "Hormones and Cancer" (Eds S. Iacobelli,
    N. Lindner and K. Griffith), Raven Press, New York,
    pp. 431-442.
15. Martini, L., Celotti, F., Massa, R. and Motta, M. (1978).
    J. Steroid Biochem. 9, 411-417.
16. Shapiro, M.I., Collu, R. and Masse, D. (1976). *Life Sci.*
    19, 1341-1346.
17. Celotti, F., Negri-Cesi, P., Limonta, P. and Melcangi,
    C. (1983). *J. Steroid Biochem.* 19, 229-234.
18. Zanisi, M., Motta, M. and Martini, L. (1973). *J. Endocr.*
    56, 315-316.
19. Martini, L., Celotti, F., Juneja, H., Motta, M. and
    Zanisi, M. (1979). *In* "Central Regulation of the
    Endocrine System" (Eds K. Fuxe, T. Hokfelt and R. Luft
    Plenum Press, New, York, pp. 273-295.
20. Imperato-Mc Ginley, J., Guerrero, L., Gautier, T. and
    Peterson, R.E. (1974). *Science* 186, 1213-1215.
21. Walsh, P.C., Madden, J.D., Harrod, M.J., Goldstein, J.L.,
    Mc Donald, P.C. and Wilson, J.D. (1974). *New Engl.
    J. Med.* 291, 944-949.
22. Peterson, R.E., Imperato-Mc Ginley, J., Gautier, T. and
    Sturla, E. (1977). *Am. J. Med.* 62, 170-191.
23. Imperato-Mc Ginley, J., Peterson, R.E., Leshin, M.,
    Griffin, J.E., Cooper, G., Draghi, S., Berenyi, M.
    and Wilson, J.D. (1980). *J. Clin. Endocr. Metab.* 50,
    15-22.
24. Zanisi, M., Motta, M. and Martini, L. (1973). *In* "The
    Endocrine Function of the Human Testis" Vol. 1, pp.
    431-436. (Eds V.H.T. James, M. Serio and L. Martini),
    Academic Press, New York.
25. Stewart-Bentley, M., Odell, W.D. and Horton, R. (1974).
    J. Clin. Endocr. Metab. 38, 545-553.
26. Verjans, H.L. and Eik-Nes, K.B. (1977). *Acta Endocr.* 84,
    842-849.
27. Odell, W.D., Swedloff, R.S., Jacobs, H.S. and Hescox, M.A
    (1973). *Endocrinology* 92, 160-165.
28. Ramirez, V.D. and McCann, S.M. (1965). *Endocrinology*
    74, 412-417.

29. Davidson, J.M. and Smith, E.R. (1967). *In* "Hormonal Steroids" (Eds L. Martini, F. Fraschini and M. Motta), pp. 805-813. Excerpta Medica, Amsterdam.
30. Negro-Vilar, A., Krulich, L. and McCann, S.M. (1973). *Endocrinology* 93, 660-664.
31. Nazian, S.J. and Mahesh, V.S. (1979). *Biol. Reprod.* 21, 465-471.
32. Massa, R., Justo, S. and Martini, L. (1975). *J. Steroid Biochem.* 6, 567-571.
33. Denef, C., Magnus, C. and McEwen, B.S. (1974). *Endocrinology* 94, 1265-1274.

HYPOTHALAMIC CONTROL OF GONADOTROPIN SECRETION

Ludwig Wildt and Gerhard Leyendecker

*Department of Obstetrics and Gynecology
University of Bonn
53 Bonn-Venusberg, FRG*

INTRODUCTION

The concept that the brain controls anterior pituitary
and ovarian function and that gonadal hormones, in turn, regulate pituitary gonadotropin secretion via negative and positive feedback loops has evolved from the pioneering work
performed by Harris and Hohlweg & Junkmann more than four decades ago and withstood the test of time. More recently, experiments in the rhesus monkey by Knobil and his colleagues
(1,2,3) and studies in women suffering from hypothalamic
amenorrhea (4,5,6) have provided new insights into the functioning of the hypothalamo-pituitary-ovarian-axis, which came
to be viewed as a system critically dependent upon pulsatile
signals delivered at an appropriate frequency and amplitude
from the hypothalamus. The following chapter represents a
brief summary of findings pertinent in this regard.

CENTRAL NERVOUS SYSTEM CONTROL OF GONADOTROPIN SECRETION

The secretion of gonadotropic hormones from the pituitary
gland is a rythmic, pulsatile phenomenon. This has first been
recognized in the ovariectomized rhesus monkey and subsequently in other species, including man (7,8,9). Because of its
characteristic frequency in the monkey, the term "circhoral
secretion" has been coined to characterize this secretory
mode (7).

Pulsatile release of gonadotropins appears to be the consequence of pulses of GnRH discharged into the pituitary portal circulation. This view is supported by the direct observation of pulses of GnRH in the pituitary portal effluent of

DOPAMINE AND NEUROENDOCRINE
ACTIVE SUBSTANCES
ISBN 0 12 209045 4

monkeys and by the demonstration that antisera against GnRH
block pulsatile gonadotropin release (10,11). The intermittent secretion of GnRH appears to be the consequence of a
synchronous discharge of GnRH-containing neurons, activated
by some neuronal pulse-generator or oscillator (2,3). This
was suggested by the earlier observation that neuroactive
drugs interrupt pulsatile LH secretion and substantiated by
the results of recordings of multiunit-activity in the area
of the arcuate nucleus, which have shown striking correlation
between electrical activity and the initiation of LH pulses
(3).

In the rhesus monkey, the circhoral oscillator which directs pulsatile GnRH release must reside within the mediobasal hypothalamus (MBH), since complete isolation of this
area from the remainder of the brain does not interfere with
pulsatile gonadotropin secretion (12). Bilateral destruction
of the arcuate nucleus within the MBH by radiofrequency lesions completely abolished gonadotropin secretion. This nucleus therefore appears to contain the neuronal elements directing pulsatile GnRH release and to mediate hypothalamic
control of gonadotropin secretion (2,13).

The physiologic significance of pulsatile gonadotropin
release did not become apparent until attempts were made to
restore gonadotropin secretion in ovariectomized monkeys with
hypothalamic lesions by the administration of exogenous GnRH.
While continuous administration of the decapeptide was able
to induce an initial increase in circulating LH and FSH levels, it failed invariably to sustain this increment. When,
however, continuous infusion was replaced by intermittent administration, consisting of one pulse per hour, thus mimicking the physiological frequency of endogenous GnRH release,
a sustained increment of LH and FSH levels could be achieved.
Moreover, a shift from pulsatile to continuous mode of infusion promptly inhibited previously reestablished gonadotropin
secretion (14). It was concluded, therefore, that the function of the hypothalamic control system that directs gonadotropin secretion is obligatorily intermittent and that the
pattern, and not the amount of GnRH delivered to the pituitary is of critical importance for the maintenance of gonadotropin secretion (2,3,14).

In this context, frequency of hypothalamic GnRH secretion
appears to play a much more important role than amplitude.
This was concluded from the results of experiments in which
the effects of different frequencies and amplitudes of GnRH
pulses on gonadotropin secretion were examined in ovariectomized lesioned monkeys (15). Increasing the frequency over
one pulse per hour led to a decline of circulating gonadotro-

pin levels while 5 pulses per hour completely abolished gonadotropin secretion in a manner similar to that observed during
constant infusion. Decreasing the frequency of GnRH pulses
from one pulse per hour to one pulse every three hours, on
the other hand, was followed by a decline of LH levels and an
increase of FSH concentrations, resulting in a dramatic
change of the FSH/LH ratio (15).

The decline of plasma gonadotropins observed at high frequency stimulation may be related to the effect of desensitization or down-regulation, while the change of the FSH/LH
ratio observed during slow frequency stimulation can be explained by an increase of the pituitary response to GnRH and
by the different disappearance times of FSH and LH from the
circulation. The increase in size of the LH-bolus is more
than matched by the time available for its disappearance.
This is not the case for FSH, permitting this glycoprotein to
accumulate in the circulation. Therefore, relatively small
changes in frequency of hypophysiotropic stimulation not only
alter the concentrations of LH and FSH, but also have major
effects on their relative proportions. In contrast, major
changes in amplitude of GnRH pulses have but minor regulatory
potential. Increasing the amplitude of GnRH pulses tenfold
had no effect on LH levels but slightly inhibited FSH secretion. Decreasing the amplitude tenfold completely abolished
gonadotropin secretion while reduction to one half of the
standard pulse amplitude produced erratically fluctuating LH
and FSH levels (15).

CONTROL OF GONADOTROPIN SECRETION DURING THE MENSTRUAL CYCLE

Amplitude and frequency of pulsatile gonadotropin secretion during the menstrual cycle are modulated by ovarian
steroids. This is particularly apparent during the human menstrual cycle, where pulses of LH can readily be observed.
Earlier studies have established that the follicular phase of
the cycle is characterized by high frequency, low amplitude
pulses while during the luteal phase low frequency, high amplitude pulses prevail (8,9). The temporal aspects of this
changing pattern of pulsatile gonadotropin secretion have been
examined recently in women at 2-4 day intervals during different phases of the menstrual cycle or daily during the midcycle surge (6,16,17). Frequency of LH pulses declined pro-
gressively during the luteal phase, reaching a nadir immediately before onset of the menstruation while pulse amplitude
appeared to increase during this time. Within the first days
following onset of menstruation, pulse frequency increased
dramatically and reached a stable plateau after 4 to 6 days.

This was associated with a decrease in pulse amplitude. No
further increase of LH pulse frequency was observed during
the midcycle surge, but a dramatic increase of pulse amplitude occurred at this time.

The changes in frequency of pulsatile LH secretion observed during the cycle are the consequence of the changing
titers of progesterone produced by the *corpus luteum* (6,16,
18,19). In this context, progesterone appears to reduce pulse
frequency in a primarily time-dependent manner, since the
lowest frequency is observed immediately before onset of menstruation, at a time when progesterone has surpassed peak
levels in the circulation (6,16). Estradiol levels do not
change significantly around menstruation, and the increase in
pulse frequency observed during the early follicular phase
may therefore be viewed as a consequence of withdrawal of the
inhibitory action of progesterone on the activity of the hypothalamic pulse generator directing gonadotropin secretion.
In contrast, amplitude of the LH pulses appears to be primarily controlled by estradiol (2,18).

The overall pattern of gonadotropin secretion during the
menstrual cycle, low, tonic secretion during the follicular
and luteal phase, interrupted by a massive discharge at midcycle has shown to be the resultant of concentration dependent inhibitory and stimulatory actions of ovarian estradiol
(1,5,20). Progesterone, secreted from the dominant follicle
immediately before ovulation, appears to enhance the stimulatory action of estradiol (5,20), while the elevated levels
of this steroid produced by the *corpus luteum* completely
block this action of estrogen (1).

Estradiol and progesterone could modulate gonadotropin secretion by acting at the hypothalamus, the pituitary gland
or at both of these sites. Considerable effort has been de-
voted to the elucidation of the site(s) at which estradiol
exerts its inhibitory and stimulatory actions on gonadotropin
secretion. Compelling evidence in favor of a pituitary site
of action has been provided by Knobil and his colleagues (2,
21). In experiments using ovariectomized monkeys with hypothalamic lesions, gonadotropin secretion was reestablished
by the intermittent administration of GnRH. When prelesion
control levels were reached, an increment in circulating
estradiol first inhibited gonadotropin secretion. This was
followed by a massive discharge of LH and FSH which was indistinguishable from that observed in monkeys with intact
central nervous system. Since this occurred in the presence
of an unvarying pulsatile GnRH replacement regimen, it was
concluded that estradiol exerts its feedback actions at the
level of the pituitary gland and that changes in hypothalamic

GnRH secretion are not necessary in this regard (2,21).

The additional observation that normal ovulatory menstrual cycles could be induced in animals with hypothalamic lesions, but intact ovaries, by applying the same unvarying pulsatile GnRH replacement regimen, has led to the conclusion, that hypothalamic GnRH secretion plays an obligatory, but only permissive role in the control system that governs the menstrual cycle of the rhesus monkey, and that gonadotropin secretion during the cycle is controlled by ovarian estrogen acting directly at the pituitary gland (2,22).

Estradiol could exert its stimulatory effects on gonadotropin secretion either by sensitizing the pituitary to an unvarying, pulsatile GnRH stimulus or by activating some other secretory mechanism. The second of these possibilities is supported by the results of experiments, in which estradiol was injected in castrated lesioned monkeys at various times after discontinuation of GnRH infusion. Discharges of LH and FSH could be induced when the steroid was injected up to 48 hours after termination of GnRH infusion, but not thereafter (23). These observations are consonant with the report by Ferin and colleagues that estrogen can induce gonadotropin discharges when administered shortly after pituitary stalk section (24) and suggests, that the steroid itself can act as a releasing hormone, when the pituitary is adequately prepared by GnRH. These findings also explain the earlier observation, that inhibition of endogenous GnRH secretion by neuroactive drugs as well as its neutralization by the acute administration of antiserum against the decapeptide were unable to block the positive feedback actions of estradiol (1,11).

In contrast to the pituitary site of action of estradiol, the progesterone blockade of estradiol induced gonadotropin discharges must be exerted at the central nervous system, since increments in circulating progesterone levels that block estrogen induced gonadotropin discharges in intact monkeys failed to do so in animals with hypothalamic lesions on GnRH replacement (25). Further experiments suggest that the blocking action of progesterone is not effected by an interruption of GnRH release, but appears to be caused by the release on an inhibitory agent from the hypothalamus (26). The facilitatory action of progesterone, on the other hand, seems to be exerted at the pituitary gland since estrogen-induced gonadotropin discharges were advanced in time during progesterone treatment of lesioned monkeys on GnRH replacement (25).

PULSATILE GONADOTROPIN SECRETION IN WOMEN WITH HYPOTHALAMIC
AMENORRHEA

Similar to monkeys with hypothalamic lesions that abolish
endogenous GnRH production and pulsatile gonadotropin secretion, a variety of circumstances that compromise normal ovarian function in women are characterized by the absence or
the severe reduction of pulsatile gonadotropin release. Since
the common final defect in those patients appears to be a
reduction of hypothalamic GnRH secretion, their condition is
referred to as "hypothalamic amenorrhea", a term coined by
Klinefelter to define amenorrhea of suprapituitary origin.
Based on studies in amenorrheic patients, prepuberal subjects and prepuberal monkeys, the view has been advanced that
hypothalamic amenorrhea represents a pathophysiological *con-
tinuum* which reflects a gliding scale of impairment of hypothalamic GnRH secretion (4,27). It was furthermore proposed
that the extent of this impairment can be assessed by the
response to gestagen, clomiphene and single bolus administration of GnRH. This concept has been substantiated by examin-
ing the pulsatile pattern of gonadotropin secretion in women
suffering from this disorder (6).
In the most severe form of hypothalamic amenorrhea, gonadotropin secretion was found to be compromised to an extent
similar to that observed in lesioned monkeys and no evidence
for pulsatile secretion of gonadotropins was found. In most
patients suffering from hypothalamic amenorrhea, however,
pulsatile gonadotropin secretion could still be observed and
frequency and amplitude of LH pulses increased with decreasing grades and severity of the disorder. In the more severe
grades, this increase in pulsatile LH secretion became only
apparent during sleep. In less severe grades, it extended
over the whole 24 hours day and reached, with respect to frequency, values comparable to that observed during the early
follicular phase of the cycle. Amplitude of the LH pulses,
however, always remained lower than in ovulating women. This
pattern is similar to that observed during the course of normal puberty, and hypothalamic amenorrhea may therefore be
viewed as a regression into puberty or as an arrest of pubertal development (4,6,27); (Fig. 1). A graded classification
of hypothalamic amenorrhea based on various tests of central
responsiveness to various *stimuli* is presented elsewhere in
this volume (see Leyendecker and Wildt, page 216).
That absence or reduction of GnRH secretion is indeed
cause of hypothalamic amenorrhea is strongly suggested by
the demonstration, that, similar to monkeys with hypothalamic

lesions, normal menstrual cycles resulting in ovulation, *cor-pus luteum* formation and eventually pregnancy could be induced in such patients by the chronic intermittent administration of an unvarying amount of GnRH (5,27,28,29).

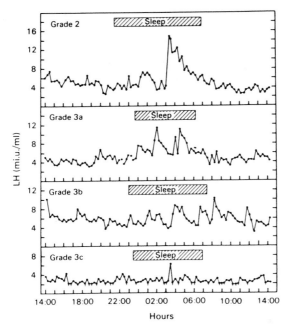

Fig. 1. 24 hour pulsatile LH patterns in patients with differ-ent severity grades of hypothalamic amenorrhea. Persistence of puberal profiles in types 2 and 3a are conspicuous.

It is tempting to speculate that the reduction of LH pulse frequency and amplitude observed in those patients reflects a corresponding reduction in frequency and amplitude of hypo-thalamic GnRH secretion. That amplitude of the GnRH pulses in subjects with intact ovaries – in contrast to ovariectomized monkeys – may indeed have regulatory potential is suggested by the results of experiments, in which women suffering from identical grades of hypothalamic amenorrhea were infused with different doses of GnRH at a constant frequency, resulting in different amplitudes of GnRH pulses. With increasing ampli-tudes, higher levels of LH, FSH, estradiol and progesterone were achieved. This strongly suggests that the amplitude of the GnRH pulse can determine the magnitude of the pituitary and ovarian response by changing the setpoint of the feed-back system operating between ovary and pituitary (5,27).

The nature of the inhibitory inputs restraining the acti-vity of the hypothalamic pulse generator in hypothalamic

amenorrhea are unknown. In this context, the demonstration
that administration of the opioid antagonist naloxone to patients suffering from hypothalamic amenorrhea reinitiates and
sustains pulsatile LH release is of considerable interest
(6,30). If endogenous opioids indeed mediate the inhibitory
inputs impinging on the neuronal pulse-generator in hypothalamic amenorrhea remains to be shown.

While hypothalamic amenorrhea is characterized by a reduced frequency and amplitude of pulsatile LH secretion, the
reverse occurs in some patients suffering from hyperandroge-
nic amenorrhea. In those gonadotropin secretion profiles are
characterized by LH pulses occuring at a supraphysiologic
frequency and amplitude (6,31). Interestingly, FSH levels are
suppressed in those patients and it is tempting to speculate
that this is the consequence of a supraphysiologic frequency
of hypothalamic GnRH secretion. It is not clear, however, if
this increase in frequency and amplitude of LH secretion is
cause of this disorder or merely the consequence of a disturbance in other components of the control system that governs
gonadotropin secretion. Once established, however, this
pattern of gonadotropin secretion could sustain and further
aggravate pituitary and ovarian dysfunction.

CONCLUSIONS

The data presented in this chapter have led to a concept
of hypothalamic control of the primate ovarian cycle, which
is fundamentally different from that developed for the laboratory rodent (2,5,32). While in the rat neural mechanisms
that link chronobiological signals and steroid levels to GnRH
release play a critical role in the control of gonadotropin
secretion and the timing of ovulation, such mechanisms seem
not to be essential in the primate, including the human female. Hypothalamic GnRH secretion rather appears to be but a
permissive component of the regulatory system governing the
menstrual cycle of higher primates and gonadotropin secretion
is primarily controlled by the action of estrogen directly
at the pituitary gland. This model, which is much simpler than
that developed for the rat, has provided the basis for a new
understanding of the pathophysiology of some forms of reproductive failure. In addition, it has led directly to new therapeutic regimens for the successful treatment of some of
these disorders.

REFERENCES

1. Knobil, E. (1974). *Recent Progr. Horm. Res.* <u>30</u>, 1-46.
2. Knobil, E. (1980). *Recent Progr. Horm. Res.* <u>36</u>, 53-88.3.
3. Knobil, E. (1981). *Biol. Reprod.* <u>24</u>, 44-49.
4. Leyendecker, G. (1979). *Eur. J. Obstet. Gynecol. Reprod. Biol.* <u>9</u>, 175-186.
5. Leyendecker, G., Wildt, L. (1983). *In* "Neuroendocrine Aspects of Reproduction" (Ed. R.L. Norman). pp. 295-323. Academic Press, New York.
6. Wildt, L., Schwilden, H., Wesner, G., Roll, C., Brensing K.A., Luckhaus, J., Bähr, M., Leyendecker, G. (1983). *In* "Brain and Pituitary Peptides II" (Eds G. Leyendecker, H. Stock, L. Wildt). pp. 28-57. Karger, Basle.
7. Dierschke, D.J., Bhattacharya, A.N., Atkinson, L.E., Knobil, E. (1970). *Endocrinology* <u>87</u>, 850-853.
8. Yen, S.S.C., Tsai, C.C., Naftolin, F., Vandenberg, G., Ajabor, L. (1972). *J. Clin. Endocrinol. Metab.* <u>34</u>, 671-675.
9. Santen, R.J., Bardin, C.W. (1973). *J. Clin. Invest.* <u>52</u>, 2617-2628.
10. Carmel, P.W., Araki, S., Ferin, M. (1976). *Endocrinology* <u>99</u>, 243-248.
11. McCormack, J.T., Plant, T.M., Hess, D.L., Knobil, E. (1977). *Endocrinology* <u>100</u>, 663-667.
12. Krey, L.C., Butler, W.R., Knobil, E. (1975). *Endocrinology* <u>96</u>, 1073-1087.
13. Plant, T.M., Krey, L.C., Moossy, J., McCormack, J.T., Hess, D.L., Knobil, E. (1978). *Endocrinology* <u>102</u>, 52-62.
14. Belchetz, P.E., Plant, T.M., Nakai, Y., Keogh, E.J., Knobil, E. (1978). *Science* <u>202</u>, 631-633.
15. Wildt, L., Häusler, A., Marshall, G., Hutchison, J.S., Plant, T.M., Belchetz, P.E., Knobil, E. (1981). *Endocrinology* <u>109</u>, 376-385.
16. Wildt, L., Brensing, K.A., Leyendecker, G. (1982). *Acta Endocrinol.* <u>99</u>, Suppl. 246, 82-83.
17. Wildt, L., Hebold, I., Leyendecker, G. (1983). *Acta Endocrinol.* <u>105</u>, Suppl. 264, 148.
18. Goodman, R.L., Karsch, F.J. (1980). *Endocrinology* <u>107</u>, 1286-1290.
19. Soules, M.R., Steiner, R.A., Clifton, D.K., Cohen, N.L., Aksel, S., Bremner, W.J. (1984). *J. Clin. Endocrinol. Metab.* <u>58</u>, 378-383.
20. Leyendecker, G., Wildt, L., Gips, H., Nocke, W., Plotz, E.J. (1976). *Arch. Gynäkol.* <u>221</u>, 29-45.

21. Nakai, Y., Plant, T.M., Hess, D.L., Keogh, E.J., Knobil,
    E. (1978). *Endocrinology* 102, 1008-1014.
22. Knobil, E., Plant, T.M., Wildt, L., Belchetz, P.E.,
    Marshall, G. (1980). *Science* 207, 1371-1373.
23. Wildt, L., Häusler, A., Hutchison, J.S., Marshall, G.,
    Knobil, E. (1981). *Endocrinology* 108, 2011-2013.
24. Ferin, M., Rosenblatt, H., Carmel, P.W., Antunes, J.L.,
    Vande Wiele, R.L. (1979). *Endocrinology* 104, 50-52.
25. Wildt, L., Hutchison, J.S., Marshall, G., Pohl, C.R.,
    Knobil, E. (1981). *Endocrinology* 109, 1293-1294.
26. Pohl, C.R., Richardson, D.W., Marshall, G., Knobil, E.
    (1982). *Endocrinology* 110, 1454-1455.
27. Leyendecker, G., Wildt, L. (1983). *J. Reprod. Fertil.*
    69, 397-409.
28. Leyendecker, G., Struve, T., Plotz, E.J. (1980). *Arch.
    Gynäkol.* 229, 177-190.
29. Leyendecker, G., Wildt, L., Hansmann, M. (1980). *J. Clin.
    Endocrinol. Metab.* 51, 1214-1216.
30. Quigley, M.E., Sheehan, K.L., Casper, R.F., Yen, S.S.C.
    (1980). *J. Clin. Endocrinol. Metab.* 50, 949-954.
31. Yen, S.S.C. (1980): *Clin. Endocrinol.* 12, 177-208.
32. Goodman, R.L., Knobil, E. (1981). *Neuroendocrinology*
    32, 57-63.

MECHANISM OF ACTION OF CLOMID: EFFECT ON LH PULSATILE RELEASE

E. del Pozo*, E. Polak[+], J. Alba-Lopez*,
D. Müller* and A. Guitelman[+]

* *Experimental Therapeutics Dept., Sandoz Ltd.,
Basle, Switzerland*

+ *Department of Endocrinology, Hospital Alvarez,
Buenos Aires, Argentina*

INTRODUCTION

The management of infertility, male and female, has progressed dramatically in the last two decades. The availability
of purified gonadotropins for clinical use and the characterization of the estrogen antagonist clomid as an ovulation in-
ducer have opened up a new era in reproductive endocrinology
(1, 2). More recently, the synthesis of the gonadotropin releasing factor (GnRH) has provided a new tool in the therapy
of gonadal insufficiency (3). After it was shown that luteinizing hormone (LH) is secreted by the pituitary in episodic
rather than continuous manner (4, 5) and that this secretory
rhythm was a pre-requisite for follicular maturation to occur
(6), the pulsatile administration of GnRH mimicking physiological hypothalamic activity has been successful in inducing
ovulation in amenorrheic women (7). However, excessive exogenous episodic gonadotrope stimulation can cause multiple
pregnancies (8), a phenomenon also observed with the use of
clomid (9). The accepted mechanism of action of the latter,
via blockade of central estrogenic receptors, does not explain the occurence of multiple follicular growth, which
would require enhancement of hypothalamic GnRH activity.

In an attempt to clarify this issue, plasma LH fluctuations
were measured in a group of normal male and female volunteers
subjected to central stimulation with clomid. Two women with
hypothalamic amenorrhea were also included in this study.

SUBJECTS AND METHODS

Six female and seven male normal volunteers were studied with the same protocol. All subjects had blood withdrawn at 15' intervals for 6 hours as a baseline and after intake of 50 mg clomid twice daily for 5 days in the female subjects and for 10 days in the males. Women started substance intake on day 3 of cycle.

Two amenorrheic females followed the same protocol. No sex steroids had been administered to induce vaginal bleeding in order to avoid sensitisation of hypothalamic activity, and clomid administration was started at random.

Integrated LH pulses were evaluated according to Santen (5) with some modifications. Pulse amplitude and frequency were also estimated. LH was measured in all samples, estradiol 17β or testosterone only in the last sample of the series. Cumulative values in the baseline and after treatment with both drugs were compared for significance by variance analysis.

RESULTS

Effect of clomid in normal volunteers

Results of clomid administration to normal volunteers are depicted in figure 1. There are no changes in the frequency of pulses but basal LH levels (bLH), integrated profiles (AUC) and pulse amplitude (A) measurements had increased significantly ($p<0.01$) in the male subjects when compared with basal values. The female volunteers also exhibited a definite trend towards higher values but without reaching the level of significance ($p<0.05$), possibly due to the small number of subjects studied.

TABLE I

Effect of clomid administration on basal E_2-17β and testosterone (nmol/l) in female and male volunteers

	basal	clomid
E_2-17β	0.18 ± .03	0.74 ± .12
n = 6		p < 0.01
T	15 ± 1.4	35.5 ± 4.3
n = 7		p <0.001

Basal estradiol 17β and testosterone values were significantly higher (p<0.01 and 0.001 respectively) at the end of the investigational period (Table I) as indicative of excessive gonadal stimulation.

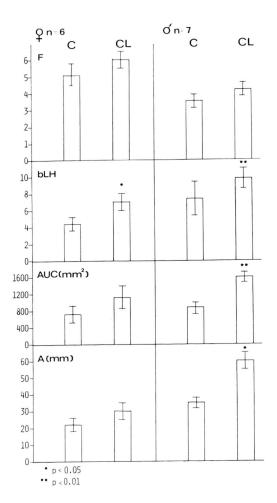

Fig. 1. Cumulative data on pulsatile LH parameters under basal conditions (C) and following the administration of clomid (Cl) to normal female and male subjects. F: frequency; bLH: basal LH; AUC: area under the curve; A: amplitude

LH and estradiol responses in hypothalamic amenorrhea

   Analysis of plasma samples in two amenorrheic women treated
with daily doses of 100 mg clomid for 5 days revealed substantial LH and estradiol increases in comparison with the baseline. Figure 2 presents the hormone profiles recorded in one
case. Basal estradiol (as E_2-17β) was below 50 pg/ml and
plasma LH exhibited average basal levels in the normal range
(7,3 mIU/ml) and fluctuations of low amplitude (1,3 mIU).
Following clomid treatment, basal LH increased to a mean of
18 mIU and larger fluctuations (2 to 9.7 mIU) were clearly
recognizable. This was reflected in estradiol pulses exceeding
75 pg above a baseline of 200 pg/ml, indicating that the ovarian follicles were responding to a biological signal. A similar response pattern was observed in the other patient.

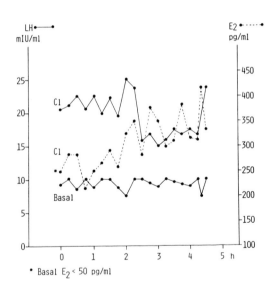

*Fig. 2. Pulsatile LH profile in a women with hypothalamic
amenorrhea following standard clomid (Cl) treatment. There is
a clear elevation of basal LH and wider pulses can be recognized. A substantial elevation of basal estradiol is conspicuous.*

COMMENTS

It is well recognized that pulsatile hypothalamic GnRH
bursts govern the episodic secretion of LH and possibly also
of FSH by the pituitary, although a periodic release of the
latter is barely demonstrable by available laboratory procedures. Recent studies have revealed that this pulsatile hypothalamic activity is subjected to a series of modulating
factors. Moreover, the gonadotrop cell response to GnRH
varies according to the frequency and intensity of such im-
pulses as reflecting up and down-regulatory mechanisms. Thus,
it has been shown not only that periodical administration
of GnRH to anovulatory females would stimulate follicular
growth and induce ovulation but that continuous infusion to
primates would reduce LH output by the pituitary (6, 10, 11).
Interestingly enough, pulsatile administration of this peptide
in increasing dosages provokes elevated gonadotrop responses
as shown by enhanced circulating LH pulses. Indeed, administration of GnRH to women under a similar regime may augment
the amplitude of plasma LH fluctuations (12) and multiple
ovulations may occur (8).

Clomiphene citrate has been characterized as an estrogen
receptor antagonist on a competitive basis (13). Indeed, this
compound was proven to be antiestrogenic when administered
in combination with ethinyl-estradiol (14). Nevertheless, the
investigation of its exact mechanism, of action pointed to
a potentiation of gonadotropin secretion (15), and specific
affinity for hypothalamic receptor sites was soon recognized,
although a simultaneous effect at the level of the pituitary
seemed likely (16, 17). After a direct action on the hypothalamus was confirmed, evidence was provided in the experimental animal that clomid treatment resulted in GnRH
release (18) and releasing-factor properties have been
attributed to this compound suggesting a trigger effect on
LH secretion (19). The sequence of events would be stimulation
of the hypothalamo-pituitary axis first to release gonadotropins via GnRH increments, followed by a biological effect on
the gonads.

The fact that, in early studies, administration of clomid
to normal women for two weeks or longer in an attempt to
inhibit ovulation was followed by prolongation of the luteal
phase (20) may reflect persistence of a particular hypothalamic secretory pattern. In the clinical situation this
eventuality is avoided by short administration of the drug.

Data reported here reveal a stimulatory action of clomid on hypothalamic activity, increasing the pulse amplitude and the area covered by the LH profiles. This effect was recorded in subjects of both sexes. No effect on the pulse timing was observed and wave frequency was not altered in subjects of both sexes. This latter finding probably suggests that this compound does not modify primary neuronal activity at the level of the medio basal hypothalamus in contrast with naloxone, a drug which increases LH puls frequency (21). The enhancement of circulating sex steroids recorded at the end of the drug administration period indicates that the secreted gonadotropins are biologically active. Considering the occurrence of this phenomenon in subjects with normal basal plasma estrogen and testosterone, hyperstimulation of the hypothalamo-gonadal axis can be assumed. Reproduction of similar hormonal profiles in two cases of normoprolactinemic amenorrhea confirms the central mechanism of action of clomid and explains the occurence of multiple ovulations in subjects exhibiting high sensitivity to this drug. These findings are in agreement with the ovarian hyperstimulation that follows excessive GnRH pulsatility by derivatives injected exogenously indicating lack of down regulation of pituitary gonadotrops at least at dosages used to date and after intermittent administration.

In conclusion, clomid administration to normal male and female subjects and to women with secondary amenorrhea estimulates hypothalamic GnRH activity as reflected in increases in LH pulsatility parameters and in enhancement of circulating gonadal steroids. These findings suggest that the primary site of action of clomid in humans is located at suprasellar level.

REFERENCES

1. Roy, S., Greenblatt, R.B., Mahesh, V.B., and Jungck, E.C. (1983). *Fertil. Steril.* 14, 575-595.
2. Borth, R., Lunenfeld, B., Riotton, G., and DeWatteville, H. (1957). *Experientia* 13, 115-117.
3. Kastin, A.J., Zarate, A., Midgley, R. Jr., Cannales, E.S., and Schally, A.V. (1971). *J. Clin. Endocrinol. Metab.* 33, 980-982.
4. Yen, S.S.C., Tsai, C.C., Naftolin, F., VandenBerg, G., and Ajabor, L. (1972). *J. Clin. Endocrinol. Metab.* 34, 671-675.

5. Santen, R.J., and Bardin, C.W. (1973). *J. Clin. Invest.* 52, 2617-2628.
6. Belchetz, P.E., Plant, T.M., Nakai, Y., Keogh, E.J., and Knobil, E. (1978). *Science* 202, 631-633.
7. Leyendecker, G., Wildt, L., and Hansmann, M. (1980). *J. Clin. Endocrinol. Metab.* 51, 1214-1216.
8. Leyendecker, G., and Wildt, L. (1982). *Geburtshilfe u. Frauenheilkd.* 42, 689-699.
9. Southam, A., and Janovski, N. (1962). *J.A.M.A.* 181, 443-445.
10. Knobil, E. (1980). *Recent Progr. Horm. Res.* 36, 53-88.
11. Knobil, E., Plant, E.T.M., Wildt, L., Belchetz, D.E., and Marshall, G. (1980). *Science* 207, 1371-1373.
12. Leyendecker, G., and Wildt, L. (1983). *J. Reprod. Fertil.* 69, 397-409.
13. Roy, S., Greenblatt, R.B., and Mahesh, V.B. (1964). *Acta Endocrinol.* 47, 645-656.
14. Greenblatt, R.B., Gambrell, R.D., Mahesh, V.B., and Scholer, H.F.L. (1971). *In* "Nobel Symposium 15. Control of Human Fertility" (Eds E. Diczfalusy and U. Borell), pp. 263-274. John Wiley & Sons, Inc., New York.
15. Smith, O.W., Smith, G.V., and Kistner, R.W. (1963). *J.A.M.A.* 184, 878-886.
16. Kato, J., Kobayashi, T., and Villee, C.A. (1968). *Endocrinology* 82, 1049-1052.
17. Miyake, A., Tasaka, K., Sakumoto, T., Kawamura, Y., Nagahara, Y., and Aono, T. (1983). *Acta Endocrinol.* 103, 289-292.
18. Baier, H., and Taubert, H.D. (1968). *Experientia* 24, 1165-1166.
19. Sato, M., and Tamada, T. (1973). *Acta Obstet. Gynecol. Jpn.* 20, 182-188.
20. Greenblatt, R.B., Roy, S., Mahesh, V.B., Barfield, W.E., and Jungck, E.C. (1962). *Am. J. Obstet. Gynecol.* 84, 900-912.
21. Moult, P.J.A., Grossman, A., Evans, J.M., Rees, L.H., and Besser, G.M. (1981). *Clin. Endocrinol.* 14, 321-324.

PROLACTIN AND LH SECRETION IN
POLYCYSTIC OVARY SYNDROME

P. Falaschi*, E. del Pozo+, M. Rosa* and A. Rocco*

*Medical Clinic V, University of Rome, 00100 Rome, Italy

+Experimental Therapeutics Department, SANDOZ LTD.,
CH-4002 Basel, Switzerland

INTRODUCTION

The polycystic ovary syndrome (PCO) represents a particular
condition of the hypothalamic-pituitary-ovarian axis clinically characterized by anovulation, hirsutism and obesity (1,2).
Its biochemical background involves a disturbance of androgen
production and metabolism leading to abnormally high synthesis
of estrogen by extra-ovarian tissues. It is generally accepted
that this excess of circulating estrogen triggers the hypothalamus which enhances GnRH pulsatile release leading to the
elevated episodic LH activity characteristic of the syndrome.
An adrenal component has been established after elevated circulating concentrations of dehydroepiandrosterone-sulfate
(DEAS), a cortical metabolite, were substantiated in patients
with PCO.
    In summary, enhanced production of DEAS, androstendione (A)
and testosterone (T) provide the substrate for peripheral synthesis of estrone (E_1) and partially estradiol (E_2) the latter
through aromatization of androgens (3-8). These circulating
sex steroids would perpetuate the vicious circle via enhanced
central LH activity and subsequent ovarian hyperstimulation
(9). Although experimental and clinical evidence has been provided for a key role of hyperandrogenism in the induction of
cystic degeneration of the ovary (10-14), recent studies have
suggested a possible function of prolactin (PRL) in the pathophysiology of PCO. Indeed, moderate hyperprolactinemia has
been described in classical PCO (15,16), presumably as a result of pituitary lactotrop hyperstimulation by circulating
estrogens.

DOPAMINE AND NEUROENDOCRINE
ACTIVE SUBSTANCES
ISBN 0 12 209045 4

The aim of the present study was to investigate the role
of PRL and its dopaminergic control mechanisms in the defec-
tive gonadotropin release characteristic of PCO.

BASAL SECRETION AND DYNAMIC BEHAVIOUR OF PROLACTIN
IN THE POLYCYSTIC OVARY SYNDROME

Forty-seven patients entered the study after the diagnosis
of PCO was established according to the *criteria* established
in Table 1.

TABLE 1

Diagnostic criteria for PCO syndrome

a) Clinical	Anovulation	
	Polycystic ovaries	
	Hirsutism	
	Normal skull x-rays	
b) Hormonal	Increased LH/FSH ratio	
	Increased plasma $T,A,DEA,DEAS,A_1$	
	Normal or reduced total E_2	

The mean basal plasma PRL was 16.2 ± 1.4 (SE) ng/ml, significantly higher ($p<0.001$) than control subjects. However,
about 30% of PCO patients exhibited values between 20 and 50
ng/ml, as frequently recorded in the so called "functional
hyperprolactinemia" (15,16).
In order to better understand the nature of the hyperprolactinemia associated with PCO, the lactotrop response to TRH
and to dopaminergic blockade with haloperidol and domperidone
was investigated. Results revealed an exaggerated response to
TRH whereas the exposure to dopamine (DA) antagonists was
followed by normal lactotrop activity (17-21). The enhanced
PRL release observed following the administration of TRH
coincided with the type of response observed in situations
of estrogen dominance such as in pregnancy, during treatment
with estroprogestins, and in male transsexuals taking estrogens (22-25). This suggests a functional origin for the hyperprolactinemia of PCO, presumably through sensitization of pituitary lactotrops by circulating estrogens. On the contrary,
the response to TRH and DA-agonists is blunted in primary
lactotrop hyperfunction (26,27). However, the possibility
that PCO-hyperprolactinemia may partially be due to an estro-

gen-mediated reduction in hypothalamic DA-activity should
also be considered. It is interesting to note that normo-pro-
lactinemic PCO patients also exhibit an exaggerated PRL-re-
sponse to TRH suggesting the presence of an increased re-
leasable   pool of PRL (17-20,28).

BROMOCRIPTINE SUPPRESSION TEST IN THE POLYCYSTIC
OVARY SYNDROME

In a previous study (9) a short-term bromocriptine (Brc)
suppression test was performed in 10 PCO patients. Doses up to
7.5 mg/day were administered for a 14 day period. Plasma PRL
decreased from 29.4±3 (SE) ng/ml to 1.9±1 (SE) ng/ml at the
end of the second week. This effect was accompanied by a
significant (p<0.001) reduction in plasma T from 107.8±7 (SE)
ng/ml to 57±3.3 (day 7) and 50.8±4.7 (SE) ng/ml (day 13)(30-
34).
Later on, this test was conducted in 13 hyper- and 24 normoprolactinemic PCO patients. The patients were subdivided in
"responders" and "non responders" on the basis of a plasma T
reduction of more than 40%. Results showed a higher incidence
in the hyperprolactinemic group (n=11,84.6%) than in the normoprolactinemic (n=10,41.6%) but it is opportune to underline
that the 41.6% positive results recorded in patients with
normal plasma PRL suggests that in a number of cases PRL is
not the main agent responsible for the blockade of ovulatory
mechanisms but rather central dopaminergic phenomena unrelated to lactotrop cell control would play a more prominent role.

CHRONIC BROMOCRIPTINE TREATMENT OF POLYCYSTIC OVARY SYNDROME

In 1974 Thorner *et al.* (35) had reported that Brc therapy
would restore ovulation in some patients with hyperprolactinemic PCO. In another study Rocco *et al.* (36) showed that daily
administration of 3.75 to 7.5 mg to 10 such patients for a
three month period could not only bring plasma PRL to the low
normal range but could also normalize previously elevated
plasma T (107±7 to 64±5 ng/ml) and E_1(9±1 ng/ml to 4.8±1 ng/
ml) levels. Estradiol was not modified by therapy. In 8 of the
women tested basal temperature adopted a biphasic pattern and
ovulation could be confirmed by plasma progesterone measurement throughout the luteal phase (36).
Later on, these studies were extended to 97 normo- and
hyperprolactinemic patients. The rate of positive responses to
Brc as expressed in a reduction of plasma T concentrations
above 40% confirmed previous findings. Thus, the acute suppression test seemed to have a predictive value as to the result

of long-term Brc therapy. In this larger group the success
rate was 91.3% for the 23 hyperprolactinemic women whereas
normoprolactinemic PCO exhibited as positive response in
39 (52.7%) out of 74 patients (33,34,37). Hirsutism improved
in 65% and 48% of the cases, respectively.

EFFECT OF BROMOCRIPTINE ON LH STIMULATION BY GnRH
AND ON LH PULSATILITY

   In order to clarify the mode of action of Brc on central
gonadotrop control, the response to standard GnRH (100 ug
i.v.) stimulation was studied in a group of 8 PCO patients,
4 hyper- and 4 normoprolactinemic, before and after 3 months
treatment with 5 mg bromocriptine daily (37). The plasma LH
profiles (Fig. 1) exhibited a significant reduction (p<0.01)
at 20 and 60 minutes unrelated to the previous plasma PRL
levels.

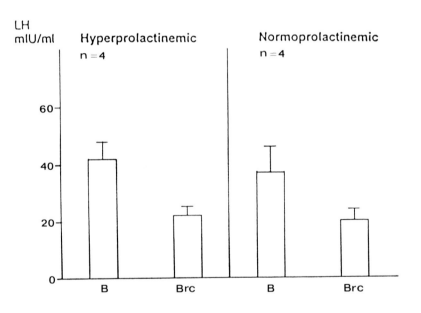

*Fig.1. LH increments following GnRH stimulation in normo- and
hyperprolactinemic women with PCO. There are no differences
between groups; (B = basal).*

Also the pulsatile LH profiles showed a clear reduction
under Brc although it was less apparent in the patients with
lower initial gonadotropin levels. Fig. 2 presents this effect
in 6 women with PCO, selected according to their responses to
the acute bromocriptine test. Again the lack of PRL dependence
is conspicuous in this group suggesting that an additional
factor may play a more important role in the reestablishment
of normal hypothalamic gonadotrop control than the circulating
lactogen levels. It can be proposed that Brc would act in this
particular condition by dampening hypothalamic activity to
bring LH control to a more physiological state. Indeed, the
integrated LH-profiles of both groups studied here showed
about the same degree of inhibition (60%, p<0.01).

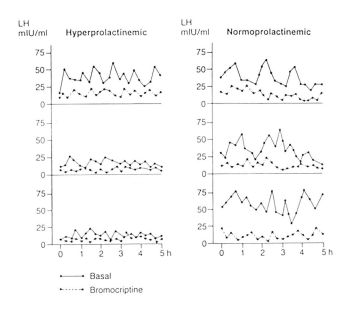

*Fig. 2. Pulsatile LH profiles of women with PCO before and
after bromocriptine treatment. The reduction in LH activity
is independent of the initial PRL levels.*

DOPAMINE AND BROMOCRIPTINE IN THE CONTROL OF LH RELEASE
IN THE POLYCYSTIC OVARY SYNDROME

How Brc exerts its favorable effect on the mechanisms governing gonadotropin release in PCO is not clearly understood.
Leblanc *et al.* (38) and Lachelin *et al.* (39) reported that

a DA infusion or the administration of Brc were able to reduce LH release in normal and in amenorrheic hyperprolactinemic women. However, DA agonists such as L-dopa, lergotrile
or apomorphine failed to modify LH plasma levels (40-43), and
Evans *et al.* (44) and Martin *et al.* (45) found no inhibitory
effect of Brc on this gonadotropin in normal or hyperprolactinemic women.

If the role of DA and dopaminergic compounds on LH secretion
in normal and hyperprolactinemic women is still debated, un-
equivocal effect has been shown in patients with PCO syndrome.
Quigley *et al.* (46) reported that a DA infusion was able to
reduce the elevated LH secretion in PCO syndrome, suggesting
that the inappropriately elevated LH release and exaggerated
LH pulses may be causally related, in part, to a reduction
of endogenous DA inhibition of LH secretory activity. Thus,
Spruce *et al.* (47) were able to show a fall in plasma LH and
T in women with PCO on long-term Brc treatment. Only patients
exhibiting such changes in their hormonal balance responded
with restoration of cyclic activity. Since the treated women
were all normoprolactinemic, a mechanism via dopaminergic LH
control could be assumed. Indeed, Faglia *et al.* (unpublished
data) have provided further evidence for a non-prolactin dependent mechanism in another series of 42 PCO patients treated
with Brc. 50% of patients responded with a fall in plasma LH
and T but these findings could not be correlated with the
basal PRL status.

The suppression of elevated pulsatile LH secretion following
chronic Brc administration in the PCO patients illustrated
here lends support to data by Quigley *et al.* (46), proposing
that the elevated and high pulsatile LH levels in those patients may result, in part, from a reduced endogenous DA inhibition of LH secretion. Brc can lower LH by increasing the
inhibitory dopaminergic tone on GnRH release. However, a direct pituitary action by reducing gonadotrop sensitivity to
hypothalamic GnRH can not be excluded, as proposed by other
authors (39,48,49).

Pituitary hyper-response to GnRH, typical of PCO, was at-
tenuated by Brc treatment. This effect may be mediated by the
same mechanism responsible for the reduction in the LH fluctuating pattern. It is interesting to observe that, in addition to PCO, increased luteotrop-cell sensitivity to GnRH is
found in other situations characterized by elevated circulating estradiol, such as in the periovulatory phase (50), but
also in primary hypogonadism (51) and in the menopause (52),
which are associated with very low estrogen production. Since
increased LH pulsatility is linked with both high and low
oestrogen levels, it is unlikely that sex steroids play a

primary role in the aetiology of PCO. This would imply a basic hypothalamic disturbance as to the cause of this condition, possibly linked to DA deficiency.

An effect of Brc at gonadal level seems unlikely. Investigations to date have failed to reveal substantial changes in ovarian or testicular function as directly related to bromocriptine, despite the presence in such tissues of specific binding sites for this drug (Martin-Perez and del Pozo, unpublished data). It seems that changes in central regulatory mechanisms are essential for Brc to show a peripheral effect.

In conclusion, the DA agonist Brc can exert a modulating effect on LH release in women with PCO. As a consequence, dampening of LH episodic activity leads to a reduction in circulating androgens and restoration of cycling activity in a number of cases.

The observed LH-inhibitory effect is recorded independently of the presence or not of hyperprolactinaemia, also thought to be mediated by decreased dopaminergic tone. This effect indicates a lack of interrelationship between dopaminergic mechanisms governing lactotrop and gonadotrop cell function, as previously pointed out by the authors (53) and elsewhere (47).

REFERENCES

1. Goldzieher, J.W. and Axelrod, L.R. (1963). *Fertil. & Steril.* 14, 631-641.
2. Yen, S.S.C. (1980). *Endocrinol.* 12, 177-207.
3. Abraham, G.E. and Charamakjian, Z.H. (1974). *Obstet. & Gynaecol.* 44, 171-175.
4. Bardin, C.W., Hemhree, W.D. and Lipsett, M.D. (1968). *J. Clin. Endocrinol. Metab.* 28, 1300-1306.
5. Horton, R. and Neisler, J. (1968). *J. Clin. Endocrinol. Metab.* 28, 479-484.
6. Judd, H.L., McPherson, R.A., Rakoff, J.S. and Yen, S.S.C. (1977). *Amer. J. Obstet. Gynaecol.* 128, 408-417.
7. Siiteri, P.K. and McDonald, P.C. (1973). *In* "Handbook of Physiology Endocrinology" (Eds R.O. Green and E. Astwood), vol. II, pp. 615-629. Amer. Physiol. Society, Washington.
8. Longcope, C. and Williams, K.I.H. (1974). *J. Clin. Endocrinol. Metab.* 38, 602-607.
9. Yen, S.S.C., Vela, P. and Rankin, J. (1970). *J. Clin. Endocrinol. Metab.* 30, 435-442.
10. Aiman, J., Nalick, R.H., Jacobs, A., Porter, J.C., Edman, C.D., Vellios, F. and McDonald, P.C. (1978). *Obstet. & Gynaecol.* 49, 695-704.

11. Benedict, P.H., Cohen, R.B., Cope, O. and Scully, R.E. (1962). *Fertil, & Steril.* <u>13</u>, 380-395.
12. Kirshner, R. and Jacobs, J. (1971). *J. Clin. Endocrinol. Metab.* <u>33</u>, 199-209.
13. Louvet, J.P., Harman, S.M., Schreiber, J.R. and Ross, G.T. (1975). *Endocrinology* <u>97</u>, 366-372.
14. Yen, S.S.C., Chaney, C. and Judd, H.L. (1976). *In* "The Endocrine Function of the Human Ovary" (Eds V.H.T. James, M. Serio and G. Giusti), pp. 373-385. Academic Press, London.
15. Falaschi, P., Frajese, G., Rocco, A., Toscano, V. and Sciarra, F. (1977). *J. Ster. Biochem.* <u>8</u>, xiii.
16. Falaschi, P., Frajese, G., Rocco, A., Toscano, V. and Sciarra, F. (1977). *Atti Giornate Endocrinologiche Pisane,* <u>I</u>, 89-92.
17. Del Pozo, E., Falaschi, P., Rocco, A., Toscano, V., Petrangeli, E., Pompei, P., Frajese, G. and Wyss, H. (1979). *In* "Abstract Book of IX World Congress of Gynaecology and Obstetrics", Tokio, p. 231.
18. Del Pozo, E. and Falaschi, P. (1980). *In* "Progress Reproductive Biology" (Eds J. Hubinot and S. Karger, Basel), vol. <u>6</u>, pp. 252-259.
19. Del Pozo, E. and Falaschi, P. (1980). *Scottish Medical J.* <u>25</u>, S89-S93.
20. Falaschi, P., del Pozo, E., Rocco, A., Toscano, V., Petrangeli, E., Pompei, P. and Frajese, G. (1980). *Obstet. & Gynaecol.* <u>55</u>, 579-582.
21. Falaschi, P., Rocco, A., Pompei, P., del Pozo, E. and Frajese, G. (1980). *In* "Abstract Book of 6th Inter. Congr. Endocrinology", Melbourne, p. 863.
22. Aono, T., Miyake, A. and Shiosi, T. (1976). *J. Clin. Endocrinol. Metab.* <u>42</u>, 696-702.
23. Del Pozo, E., Varga, L., Wyss, H., Tolis, G., Friesen, H., Wenner, R., Vetter, L. and Uettwiler, A. (1974). *J. Clin. Endocrinol. Metab.* <u>39</u>, 18-26.
24. Healy, D.L., Pepperell, R.J. and Stockdale, J. (1977). *J. Endocrinol. Metab.* <u>44</u>, 809-819.
25. Reymond, M. and Lemarchand Beraud T. (1976). *Clin. Endocrinol.* <u>5</u>, 429-436.
26. Barbarino, A., De Marinis, L., Maira, G., Menini, E. and Anile, L. (1978). *J. Clin. Endocrinol. Metab.* <u>47</u>, 1148-1151.
27. Faglia, G., Moriondo, P., Beck-Peccoz, P., Travaglini, P., Ambosi, B., Spada, A. and Nissin, M. (1980). *In* "Neuroactive Drugs in Endocrinology" (Ed. E.E. Müller) pp. 263-278. Elsevier/North Holland Biomedical Press.

28. Falaschi, P., Rocco, A., Pompei, P., del Pozo, E. and
    Frajese, G. (1979). *In* "Neuroactive Drugs in Endo-
    crinology" (Ed. E.E. Müller), Ricerca Scientifica ed
    Educazione Permanente, Suppl. 10, p.46.
29. Falaschi, P., Rocco, A., Sciarra, F., Toscano, V. and
    Frajese, G. (1979). *In* "Research and Steroids" (Eds
    A. Klopper, L. Lerner, H.J. Van der Molen and F.
    Sciarra), vol. 21, pp. 241-245. Academic Press, London.
30. Falaschi, P., Rocco, A., Frajese, G. and Conti, C. (1978).
    Triangolo XVI, 3, 66-70.
31. Falaschi, P., Frajese, G., Rocco, A., Toscano, V., Petran-
    geli, E., Sciarra, F. and Conti, C. (1978). "Atti
    XVII Congresso Nazionale Soc. Ital. Endocrinologia",
    abstract c25.
32. Falaschi, P., Rocco, A., Pompei, P., Sciarra, F. and
    Frajese, G. (1979). *J. Ster. Biochem.* 11, XIX.
33. Falaschi, P., Rocco, A., del Pozo, E. and Frajese, G.
    (1981). "Prolattina 1981", Estratti Congresso, April
    6-7, Milano.
34. Falaschi, P., Rocco, A., Bernardini, L., d'Urso, R., del
    Pozo, E., Frajese, G. and Motta, M. (1982). "Atti
    S.I.F.E.S." (in press).
35. Thorner, M.O., McNeilly, A.S., Hagan, C. and Besser, G.M.
    (1974). *Brit. Med. J.* 2, 419-422.
36. Rocco, A., Falaschi, P., Pompei, P., del Pozo, E. and
    Frajese, G. (1979). *In* "Psychoneuroendocrinology in
    Reproduction" (Eds L. Zichella and P. Pancheri),
    pp. 387-394. Elsevier/North Holland, Biomedical Press,
    Amsterdam.
37. Falaschi, P. and del Pozo, E. (1983). *In* "Lisuride and
    Other Dopamine Agonists. Basic Mechanism and Endocrine
    and Neurological Effects" (Eds D.B. Calne, R.J.
    McDonald, R. Horowski and W. Wuttke), pp. 325-330.
    Raven Press, New York.
38. Leblanc, H., Lachelin, G.C.L., Abu-Fadil, S. and Yen,
    S.S.C. (1976). *J. Clin. Endocrinol. Metab.* 43, 668-674.
39. Lachelin, G.C., Leblanc, H. and Yen, S.S.C. (1977).
    J. Clin. Endocrinol. Metab. 44, 728-732.
40. Zarate, A., Canales, E.S., Soria, J., Maneiro, P.J. and
    McGregor, C. (1973). *Neuroendocrinology* 12, 362-365.
41. Thorner, M.O., Ryan, S.M., Wass, J.A.H., Jones, A.,
    Bouloux, P., Williams, S. and Besser, G.M. (1978).
    J. Clin. Endocrinol. Metab. 47, 372-378.
42. Tolis, G.E., Pinter, E.J. and Friesen, H.G. (1975).
    Int. J. Clin. Pharmacol. 12, 281-283.
43. Lal, S., de la Vega, S.E., Sourkes, T.L. and Friesen,
    H.G. (1973). *J. Clin. Endocrinol. Metab.* 37, 719-724.

44. Evans, W.S., Rogol, A.D., MacLeod, R. and Thorner, M.O. (1980). *J. Clin. Endocrinol. Metab.* 50, 103-107.
45. Martin, W.H., Rogol, A.D., Kaiser, D.L. and Thorner, M.O. (1981). *J. Clin. Endocrinol. Metab.* 52, 650-656.
46. Quigley, M.E., Rakoff, J.S. and Yen, S.S.C. (1981). *J. Clin. Endocrinol. Metab.* 52, 231-234.
47. Spruce, B.A., Kendall-Taylor, P., Dunlop, W., Anderson, A.J., Watson, M.J., Cook, D.B. and Gray, C. (1984). *Clin. Endocrinol.* 20, 481.
48. Leebaw, W.F., Lee, L.A. and Woolf, P.D. (1978). *J. Clin. Endocrinol. Metab.* 47, 480-487.
49. Melis, G.B., Paoletti, A.M., Mais, V., Gambacciani, M., Guarneri, G., Strigini, F., Fruzetti, F. and Fioretti, P. (1981). *J. Clin. Endocrinol. Metab.* 53, 530-537.
50. Judd, S.J., Rakoff, J.S. and Yen, S.S.C. (1978). *J. Clin. Endocrinol. Metab.* 47, 494-498.
51. Siler, T.M. and Yen, S.S.C. (1973). *J. Clin. Endocrinol. Metab.* 37, 491-494.
52. Scaglia, H., Medina, M., Pinto-Ferreira, A.K., Vasquez, G., Gual, C. and Perez-Palacios, G. (1976). *Acta Endocrinol.* (Kbh) 81, 673-679.
53. Del Pozo, E., Lamberts, S.W.J., Falaschi, P. and Buchs, A. (1984). *In* "Pituitary Hyperfunction: Physiopathology and Clinical Aspects" (Eds F. Camanni and E.E. Müller), pp. 289-302. Raven Press, New York.

V. Opiates: Neuroendocrine Correlations and Pain

OPIOIDS IN THE NEUROENDOCRINE CONTROL OF THE ANTERIOR PITUITARY

E.E. Müller[*], V. Locatelli[*], S. Cella[*], C. Invitti[+],
F. Cavagnini[+] and D. Cocchi[*]

*Department of Pharmacology, University
of Milan, 20129 Milan, Italy*

+*First Medical Clinic, University
of Milan, 20122 Milan, Italy*

INTRODUCTION

Extensive research in the last 15 years has shown that in addition to classic hypothalamic regulatory hormones (RHs), e.g. TRH, LH-RH, CRF, GRF and somatostatin, a variety of other peptides exist in the central nervous system (CNS). There is little doubt that the major direct control of anterior pituitary (AP) hormone secretion is accomplished by RHs and dopamine (DA), which accounts at least partially for the prolactin-inhibiting factor (PIF) activity of the hypothalamus. However, the various neuropeptides not thought to be primarily hypophysiotropic have now been shown to affect pituitary hormone secretion, though the physiological significance of these endocrine effects is far from clear (1).

Amongst neuropeptides, endogenous opioid peptides (EOPs) have adopted a prominent role (2). Major steps in the characterization of these compounds comprise the discovery of endogenous opioid receptors (3,4); the isolation and determination of the structure of the enkephalins (5) and endorphins (6); and the finding that the physiologic hormone precursor of EOPs, e.g. proopiomelanocortin, is synthesized not only in the anterior and intermediate lobes of the pituitary, but also in neurons originating in the arcuate *nucleus* region of the mediobasal hypothalamus (MBH) (7).

Immunohistochemical studies revealed a broad distribution of peptides belonging to the EOP family throughout the CNS.

Enkephalin perikarya in the hypothalamus appear to be short
interneurons originating and terminating within the hypothalamus, but there is an extensive distribution of enkephalin-con-
taining systems throughout the whole brain and spinal cord.
In contrast, neurons containing β-END (and ACTH) are few in
numbers, are concentrated in the arcuate *nucleus* and its immediate neighbourhood and give rise to long projections reaching
as far down as the spinal cord. Peptides belonging to the proenkephalin β family (dynorphin) have also been observed in many
neurons with a distribution as wide as the enkephalin immunoreactive systems, though detailed distribution have revealed
that the dynorphin systems are separate from the enkephalin-
containing ones (8).

   The very high concentrations of the opioids in the hypothalamus suggests that they may be important in neuroendocrine
regulation, though the CNS sites for the interaction(s) between
opioids and hypophysiotropic and/or neurotransmitter neurons
are largely ignored.

   This contribution provides a brief overview of the effects
of opiates and EOPs on pituitary function and describes some
aspects of their interactions with classical neurotransmitters
in the regulation of growth hormone (GH) and prolactin (PRL)
secretion.

ACTIONS OF MORPHINE AND EOPs ON ANTERIOR PITUITARY FUNCTION

   The endocrine actions of EOPs in subprimate and primate
species resemble those of morphine (MOR); thus, we will first
discuss these effects and then relate them to the new knowledge
of the EOPs. Morphine was first reported to block ovulation
in 1955 (9). A few years later, induction of PRL release by MOR
was described, based on its ability to initiate lactation in
estrogen-primed rats (10). It was also reported to stimulate
ACTH secretion as indicated by an elevation of plasma adrenal
steroid levels (11).

   Advent of the radioimmunoassay era allowed the delineation
of the full spectrum of changes in AP hormone secretion reduced by MOR as follows: in rats it stimulates ACTH, GH and
PRL release and inhibits FSH, LH and TSH release. Some of the
effects evoked by MOR in rats are also elicited in humans, e.g
those on PRL and gonadotropin release; however, the opiate
fails to release GH in man, and suppresses instead of stimulating the pituitary-adrenal axis (12). It is of note that also
in rodents chronic MOR administration has long been known to
suppress ACTH release (13).

Although it was considered that these were pharmacological actions of MOR, it now appears likely that the opiate was interacting with opioid receptors in the brain (see below). In fact, EOPs administered systematically. or intraventricularly (I.C.V.) evoked a similar pattern of hormonal response (1). I.C.V. injection of Met-ENK, Leu-ENK, β-End all raised serum PRL and GH levels in the rat, but β-END was found to be much more effective than enkephalins (14). Also, enkephalin analogues, e.g. Met-Enk-amide, D-Ala^2-Leu^5-Enk-amide, D-Met^2-Pro^5-Enk-amide, and the enkephalin analogue FK 33-824 each stimulated PRL and GH release, and this could be blocked by the opiate receptor antagonist naloxone (NAL) (15). FK 33-824 was also shown to increase PRL and GH in human subjects. Similarly to MOR, systemic administration of Met-ENK induced a fall in serum LH but not FSH levels in male rats, while NAL blocked the inhibitory effect of Met-ENK on LH secretion. In humans, FK 33-824 significantly reduced serum LH and to a lesser extent FSH concentrations, an effect partially reversed by NAL (16).

Information relevant to the physiologic role of EOPs on AP function can be derived from studies on the effects of suppression of the intrinsic opiatergic tone by NAL. In rats, NAL lowers baseline levels of PRL response to painful stress and suckling (15). However, in humans, NAL, despite its ability to counteract the PRL-releasing effect of exogenous opioids, has little or no ability to alter basal and stimulated PRL release (17). NAL given to rats significantly increase basal serum concentrations and magnifies the preovulatory rise of both gonadotropins (18); similarly, a biphasic rise in serum LH and FSH following NAL has been reported in humans (17). In both rats (19) and humans (17) NAL alone elevated adrenal corticosteroid levels. These results taken together would implicate opiate receptors in only some aspects of the control of GH and PRL secretion in man, while the ability of NAL to increase serum levels of cortisol and LH suggests that EOPs may play a physiological role in modulating basal release of these hormones.

Mechanism of Action

Receptors. Little information is available to define the possible selectivity of receptors involved in the endocrine effects of EOPs. The existence of six different opioid receptors has been postulated including mu_1, mu_2, δ, ε, K and σ, and selective agonist interactions with each of these receptor subtypes may result in a different spectrum of pharmacological actions (2). At present the mu and δ receptors, with particular sensitivity to MOR and Leu-ENK, are best characterized. However, there is also evidence for a K receptor, whose putative endogenous ligand is dynorphin (2), and the presence in the rat *vas de-ferens* of specific β-END or ε receptors, has been suggested (20). As alluded to above the opioid antagonist NAL has been widely used in this context. However, NAL has antagonistic actions on more than one of the receptor subtypes and its utility in defining the biologic involvement of specific opioid receptors is limited. Moreover, there is evidence that NAL may under certain circumstances assume agonist properties, and at high concentrations interact with other neurotransmitter receptors (2). Opioid antagonists have recently become available with relative selectivity for mu and δ binding sites; these include the mu antagonist β-funaltrexamine (β-FNA) (22) and a δ antagonist ICI 154,129 (23). They promise to allow better delineation than NAL of receptor subtypes involved in endocrine responses. Another approach may rely on the use of different opiate alkaloids, each with differing opiate receptors affinities, and to study their effects on circulating AP hormones, in an attempt to analyze the particular receptor subtype involved in each hormonal response. The different opioid receptors allegedly involved in neuroendocrine function are reported in Table 1.

Table 1

Opioid receptors allegedly involved in neuroendocrine function

Hormone	Response	Type of Receptor	References
ACTH	↓ ↑[a]	δ , K	(37)
TSH	↓ ↑	mu , K	(37)
LH	↓	mu, δ , ε, K	(37–39)
GH	↑	δ , K	(40)
PRL	↑	mu_1, mu_2, ε , K	(37–40)

[a]The two arrows denote opposite effects in the rat and man.

It can be seen that no definitive conclusions can be drawn from these preliminary studies, since for each AP hormone more than one receptor subtype appears to be involved. Conceivably, differences in experimental conditions and/or species may underlie this pattern. Certainly, synthesis and characterization of more specific opiate ligands will allow a more precise delineation of receptor subtypes.

Neurotransmitters. It is generally agreed that opiates and EOPs do not act directly on the AP but via the CNS (15). In brief, no effect on the *in vitro* release of AP hormones is seen when enkephalin analogues or MOR are added to an incubation medium containing normal rat AP tissue; in addition, it has been shown that the EOPs do not interfere *in vivo* with the action of LHRH on LH release or TRH on TSH release. Conversely, direct instillation of MOR or β-END in the rat MBH provokes changes in AP hormone release similar to those obtained with I.C.V. or systematic injection of these compounds (24). *In vitro*, opiates do not alter the spontaneous release of RH's (e.g. somatostatin, LHRH) from MBH slices, but appear to inhibit the K^+-stimulated hormone release via specific receptors, probably by modulating Ca^{++} entry through voltage dependent Ca^{++} channels (25). Though this interaction may account e.g. for the changes in pituitary GH induced by EOPs, *in vivo* investigations showing that somatostatin antiserum did not interfere with the ability of opioids to stimulate GH release in the rat (26) would imply an action exerted via stimulation of GRF activity. It cannot be excluded that both RHs of GH release are involved in opioid modulation, possibly with different receptor subtypes (see above).

Parallel to the interactions of EOPs and several neurotransmitters in different brain areas and in the peripheral nervous system (27) is their functional interaction with a host of neurotransmitters involved in the neural control of AP function. Briefly, evidence obtained mainly with the use of MOR, enkephalin analogues e.g. FK 33-824 and, conversely, NAL, would indicate that the opposing effect on TSH secretion, inhibitory in rodents, stimulatory in humans, occurs via stimulation or inhibition, respectively, of DA function; inhibition of gonadotropin release takes place through suppression of NE function, while the PRL-releasing effect is mediated by an impairment of DA turnover. A great variety of neurotransmitters, including NE, ACh, H, DA and GABA, have been implicated in the GH-releasing effect of EOPs, while for the secretion of ACTH inhibition of an excitatory NE pathway has been postulated (28).

In view of the important role played by α-adrenergic mechanism(s) in stimulating GH secretion, attention has been focused on possible mediation of the effect of MOR and opioids on GH release by adrenergic neurotransmission. Controversial findings have been reported in this context: in rats the participation of brain NE has been either advocated (29) or refuted (30) in experiments with inhibitors of NE function. In dogs, a species more similar to humans than rats regarding GH regulation, pretreatment with yohimbine, a selective α_2-receptor antagonist, but not with phentolamine, a non-specific α-adrenergic antagonist, inhibited the rise in GH levels induced by FK 33-824 (31, and author's unpublished results). More recently, the inability of phentolamine to alter the GH-releasing effect of FK 33-824 has been confirmed in humans (32).

Though the evidence reported so far implicates mainly TIDA function in mediating the PRL-releasing effect of opioids (see above), other neurotransmitters, e.g. 5-HT, may be involved (33). Some recent findings of ours also point in this direction. Consistent with DA-mediated action is the inability of FK 33-824 to elicit a rise in plasma PRL in rats bearing an estrogen-induced prolactinoma, in which there is evidence for a reduced TIDA function (34). However, in spite of the impaired TIDA neuronal function of aged hyperprolactinemic female rats (35), they exhibit a greater PRL response to FK 33-824 than young controls (author's unpublished results), a finding that may be related to the enhanced 5-HT function present in aged rats(36).

CONCLUSIONS

There is no doubt that EOPs stimulate PRL and GH release in both rats and humans, though only in rats is there good evidence for the existence of a tonic EOP input on unstimulated hormone release. On the other hand, there is evidence that EOPs in both rats and humans play a physiologic role in modulating basal release of LH and adrenocorticotropin.

The endocrine effects of EOPs occur via the CNS, likely the hypothalamus, are mediated by a constellation of receptor subtypes e.g. mu_1, mu_2, δ, ε, K and , and involve a functional interaction with brain neurotransmitters, especially DA and NE. However, precise characterization of receptor subtype(s) involved in the secretion of each AP hormone is lacking and the CNS sites of EOP-neurotransmitter interactions and the modes of this communication are poorly understood.

ACKNOWLEDGEMENTS

The authors are grateful to Miss Maria Lupo for secretarial help.

REFERENCES

1. Mc Cann, S.M. (1982). *In* "Neuroendocrine Perspectives"
    (Eds E.E. Müller and R.M. Mac Leod) Vol.1, pp. 1-22.
    Elsevier, Amsterdam.
2. Herz, A. (1984). *In* "Central and Peripheral Endorphins"
    (Eds E.E. Müller. and E.R. Genazzani , Raven Press,
    New York.
3. Goldstein, A., Lowney, L.I. and Pal, B.K. (1971). *Proc.*
    Natl. Acad. Sci. USA 68, 1742-1747.
4. Pert, C.B. and Snyder, S.H. (1973). *Science* 179, 41-46.
5. Hughes, J., Smith, T.W., Kosterlitz, H.W., Fothergill,
    L.A., Morgan, B.A. and Morris H.R. (1975). *Nature*
    258, 577-579.
6. Li, C.H. and Chung, D. (1976). *Proc. Natl. Acad. Sci. USA*
    73, 1145-1148.
7. Watson, S.J. and Akil, H. (1981). *In* "Neurosecretion and
    Brain Peptides" (Eds J.B. Martin, S. Reichlin and
    K.L. Bick), pp. 77-86. Raven Press, New York.
8. Hökfelt, T., Vincent, S., Dalsgaard, C.J., Herrera-Mars-
    chitz, M. and Terenius, L. (1984). *In* "Central and
    Peripheral Endorphins" (Eds E.E. Müller and A.R.
    Genazzani), Raven Press, New York.
9. Barraclough, C.A. and Sawyer, C.H. (1955). *Endocrinology*
    57, 329-337.
10. Meites, J. (1962). *In* "Pharmacological Control of Release
    of Hormones Including Diabetic Drugs" pp. 151-180
    (Ed. R. Guillemin), Pergamon Press, London.
11. George, R. (1971). *In* "Narcotics" pp. 283-299 (Ed. D.H.
    Klist), Plenum Press, New York.
12. Tolis, G., Hickey, J. and Guyda, H. (1975). *J. Clin.*
    Endocrinol. Metab. 41, 797-800.
13. Briggs, F.N. and Munson, P.L. (1955). *Endocrinology* 57,
    205-219.
14. Dupont, A., Cusan, L., Labrie, F., Coy, D.H. and Li, C.H.
    (1977). *Biochem. Biophys. Res. Commun.* 75, 76-82.
15. Van Vugt, D.A. and Meites, J. (1980). *Fed. Proc.* 39,
    2533-2538.
16. Stubbs, W.A., Jones, A., Edwards, C.R.W., Delitala, G.,
    Jeffcoate, W.J., Ratter, S.J. and Besser, G.M. (1978).
    Lancet 2, 1225-1227.
17. Morley, J.E., Baranetsky, N.G., Wingert, D., Carlson, H.E.,
    Hershman, J.M., Melmed, S., Levin, S.R., Jameson, K.R.,
    Weitzman, R., Chang, R.J. and Varner, A.A. (1980).
    J. Clin. Endocrinol. Metab. 50, 251-257.

18. Ieiri, T., Chen, H.T., Campbell, G.A. and Meites, J. (1980). *Endocrinology* 106, 1568-1570.
19. Ferri, S., Spampinato, S., Arrigo-Reina, R., Stanzani, S., Occhiuto, F. and Costa, G. (1980). *Neuroendocr. Lett.* 2, 129-132.
20. Wuster, W., Schultz,.R. and Herz, A. (1981). *Biochem. Pharmac.* 36, 1883-1887.
21. Sawynok, J., Pinsky, C. and La Bella, F.S. (1979). *Life Sci.* 25, 1621-1632.
22. Takemori, A.E., Larson, D.L. and Portoghese, P.S. (1981). *Europ. J. Pharmac.* 70, 445-451.
23. Shaw, J.S., Miller, L., Turnbull, M.J., Gormley, J.J. and Morley, J.S. (1982). *Life Sci.* 31, 59-62.
24. Grandison, L. and Guidotti, A. (1977). *Nature* 250, 357-359.
25. Drouva, S.V., Epelbaum, J., Tapia-Arancibia, L., Laplante, E. and Kordon, C. (1981). *Neuroendocrinology* 32, 162-167.
26. Dupont, A., Barden, N., Cusan, L., Merand, Y., Labrie, F. and Vaudry, H. (1980). *Fed. Proc.* 39, 2545-2550.
27. Holaday, J.W. and Loh, H.H. (1981). *In* "Hormonal Protein and Peptides" vol. 10, pp. 203-291 (Ed. C.H.), Academic Press, New York.
28. Grossman, A. and Besser, G.M. (1982). *Clin. Endocrinol.* 17, 277-290.
29. Katakami, H., Kato, Y., Matsushita, N., Shimatsu, A. and Imura, H. (1981). *Endocrinology* 109, 1033-1036.
30. Shaar, C.J. and Clemens, J.A. (1980). *Fed. Proc.* 39, 2539-2543.
31. Casanueva, F., Betti, R., Cocchi, D., Chieli, T., Mantegaza, P. and Müller, E.E. (1981). *Endocrinology* 108, 157-163.
32. Penalva, A., Villanueva, L., Casanueva, F., Cavagnini, F., Gomez-Pan, A. and Müller, E.E. (1983). *Psychopharmacology* 80, 120-124.
33. Spampinato, S., Locatelli, V., Cocchi, D., Vicentini, L., Bajusz, S., Ferri, S. and Müller, E.E. (1979). *Endocrinology.* 105, 163-170.
34. Casanueva, F., Cocchi, D., Locatelli, V., Flauto, C., Zanbotti, F., Bestetti, G., Rossi, G.L. and Müller, E.E. (1982). *Endocrinology* 110, 590-599.
35. Gudelsky, G.A., Nansel, D.D. and Porter, J.C. (1981). *Brain Res.* 205, 446-450.
36. Simpkins, J.W., Mueller, G.P., Huang, H.H. and Meites, J. (1977). *Endocrinology* 100, 1672,1678.
37. Delitala, G., Grossman, A. and Besser, M. (1983). *Neuroendocrinology* 37, 275-279.

38. Holaday, J.W. and Tortella, F.C. (1984). *In* "Central
    and Peripheral Endorphins" (Eds E.E. Müller and
    A.R. Genazzani), Raven Press (in press).
39. Pfeiffer, D.G., Pfeiffer, A., Shimohigashi, Y., Merriam,
    G.R. and Loriaux, D.L. (1983). *Peptides* 4, 647-649.
40. Krulich, L. and Koenig, J.I. (1984). *In* "The Opioid
    Modulation of the Endocrine Function" (Eds M. Serio,
    G. Delitala and L. Martini), Raven Press (in press).

EFFECT OF OPIATES ON THE PITUITARY-GONADAL AXIS IN MALES

Jack H. Mendelson and Nancy K. Mello

Alcohol and Drug Abuse Research Center
Harvard Medical School-McLean Hospital
115 Mill Street, Belmont, MA 02178, U.S.A.

INTRODUCTION

Chronic opiate self-administration has been reported to
be associated with diminished sexual behavior in men (19).
Opiate dependent males frequently report decreased libido and
impaired sexual performance which is characterized primarily
by impotence (16). However, following cessation of opiate use
there is often prompt resumption of sexual drive and behavior (16).

Opiate agonist drugs suppress pituitary gonadotrophins
(e.g. luteinizing hormone, LH) and gonadal steroids (e.g.
testosterone) in humans (1,3,5,14) and in animals (2). Although the mechanism of action is unknown, opiates appear to
inhibit gonadotrophin releasing hormones in the hypothalamus
(2). Tolerance to opiate induced suppression of pituitary gonadal hormones in human males occurs during chronic drug administration (10). However, complete tolerance to opiate induced changes in levels of pituitary gonadal hormones in humans has not been observed (10). Pituitary gonadal hormones
return to normal levels following opiate abstinence in adult
males (7,9).

A number of social and cultural factors, including heroin
availability, influence the age at which heroin use begins.
In the United States, most men who chronically self-adminis-
ter heroin initiate this behavior after puberty, during their
late teens or early twenties. In areas of the world where
pure heroin is relatively inexpensive and easily procured
(e.g. Hong Kong), young men often begin heroin self-administration relatively early, between ages 11 to 15, a period before and during puberty. The temporal coincidence of heroin
use and sexual maturation appears to involve diametrically
opposite hormonal processes. The onset of puberty and psychosexual maturation in males is associates with increased se-

DOPAMINE AND NEUROENDOCRINE
ACTIVE SUBSTANCES
ISBN 0 12 209045 4

cretion of pituitary gonadotrophins (LH) and testosterone
whereas acute and chronic administration of heroin suppresses
secretion of these hormones. These data suggested that chronic heroin use during early, middle or late puberty might impair normal psychosexual growth and development.

The purpose of this investigation was to measure pituitary
gonadal hormone levels and assess psychosexual development
in a group of young men who initiated chronic heroin self-
administration during their early teens. These subjects had
abstained from drug use for at least 6 months prior to the
study, therefore acute opiate effects could not influence hormonal data obtained. The opiate abstinent subjects were compared with 2 male control groups of similar age with respect
to pituitary gonadal hormone levels and psychosexual growth
and development. The drug-free control group had never used
heroin or other opiates. A second control group had initiated
heroin self-administration after puberty and continued to use
heroin actively at the time of the study.

METHODS

Forty-three healthy adult men provided informed consent
for participation in these studies. All subjects were recruit-
ed through the Society for the Aid and Rehabilitation of Drug
Addicts (SARDA) in Hong Kong. Subjects were paid the equivalent of 10 U.S. dollars for participation in an interview and
providing blood and urine samples as described below.

Seventeen active heroin users (mean age=21.3) began to use
heroin after puberty at an average age of 17. These subjects
took their last heroin dose an average of 5.5 hrs. before
blood sampling in this study. Sixteen heroin abstinent subjects (mean age=20.8) began heroin use at an average age of
13.5 years. This group had been drug free for an average of
278 days before blood sampling. Ten normal controls (mean
age=22.8) had never used heroin.

The interviews were conducted by an experienced bilingual
interviewer at a time when the investigators were also present
Since many of the active and former heroin users were not lit-
erate in Cantonese, all subjects were interviewed in a Cantonese dialect and responses were immediately recorded on standardized data forms.

Subjects were given a standardized structured interview,
designed to assess current sexual behavior patterns, including general interest in sexual activity (all males were hetero
sexual); ability to become sexually aroused during foreplay;
and overall frequency of sexual behavior, including intercourse. The structured interview also explored the effects

of heroin self-administration on sexual interest and desire
as well as heroin effects on ability to achieve and maintain
an erection and attain ejaculation. The interview included
questions about the onset of recurrent morning penile erections and nocturnal emissions in an effort to determine the
temporal course of puberty. A history of duration of heroin
use, periods of abstinence, patterns of drug self-administration as well as a medical, legal and social history were also
obtained.

Each subject was given a complete medical examination which
included assessment of development of bone and muscle structure, facial, axillary and public hair growth and development
of external genitalia. A urine specimen was obtained at the
time of the interview for analysis of opiates, barbiturates,
stimulants and sedative hypnotic drugs. A 15 ml blood sample
was obtained by venepuncture. The blood was centrifuged immediately and the plasma was separated and frozen. Frozen plasma
samples were shipped in dry ice via air express to the United
States for analysis.

Luteinizing hormone (LH) and testosterone plasma levels
were determined by radioimmunoassay procedures. Analysis of
plasma samples for testosterone were carried out by a double
antibody radioimmunoassay modified from a procedure used for
protein hormones by Niswender *et al.* (17) and discussed in
detail in previous publications (11,12,13). Plasma LH concentrations were measured with a double antibody method similar
to that described by Midgley (15). Statistical analysis of
data were carried out with a nonparametric procedure (Mann-
Whitney U Test).

RESULTS

All subjects reported that heroin self-administration was
associated with decreased sexual desire and difficulty in
initiating and maintaining an erection during heterosexual
intercourse. All subjects also reported that during periods
of heroin abstinence, sexual interest and performance improved significantly. However, most subjects reported a low
to moderate degree of sexual interest and arousal, independent
of heroin abstinence or use.

Heroin addicts sometimes assert that opiates enhance sexual
performance insofar as time to ejaculation is decreased (7,9).
Similar claims have been made for alcohol intoxication (18,20),
which also suppresses testosterone levels (6,8). However,
among this group of former and current users only 10 individuals or 23 percent associated heroin with improved sexual performance.

Physical examination of all subjects revealed that they
were in good health. No subject in either the heroin or abstinent group showed any signs of impaired muscle growth, re-
tarded development, distribution of normal male hair growth
patterns, or development of external genitalia. There were
no significant differences in body fat distribution, height
or weight between controls, active heroin users and abstinent
subjects.

The time course of pubertal development was well within
the normal range established for adolescent males (4). Moreover, there were no significant differences betwenn the 3
groups in age of onset morning penile erections or nocturnal emissions. This similarity is interesting since the abstinent group had initiated heroin use 6 months prior to or
following the onset of morning penile erections and 6 months
prior to nocturnal emissions. These data suggest that initiation of heroin use before and during the emergence of morning
penile erections did not impair this phase of pubertal development.

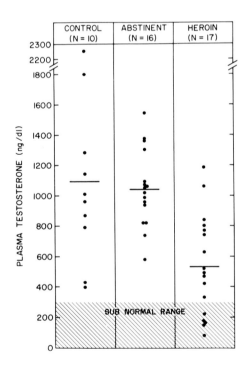

*Fig. 1. Plasma testosterone (ng/dl) for control, abstinent
and heroin using subjects.*

Urine specimens of all heroin users showed the presence
of morphine. No other drugs were present in the samples.
Urine samples from the abstinent subjects revealed no morphine
or any other drug. There were no false negative reports by
the active heroin using group and no false positive reports
by the abstinent group.

No subjects reported use of stimulant, depressant or psy-
chedelic drugs. No subject reported regular use of alcohol
except for an occasional beer. All subjects (including controls) smoked between 1 to 2 packs of cigarettes per day.

Plasma testosterone levels for the 3 groups of subjects
are shown in Fig. 1. There were no significant differences
between plasma testosterone levels in the control and abstinent subjects. Testosterone levels were significantly depressed (p<0.01) in the heroin using group and 5 to 17 subjects had plasma testosterone levels in the subnormal range.

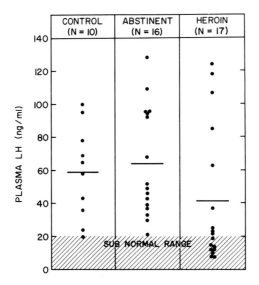

*Fig. 2. Plasma luteinizing hormone (ng/ml) for control, ab-
stinent and heroin using subjects.*

Plasma luteinizing hormone levels are presented for the 3
groups of subjects in Fig. 2. There were no significant differences between the control and abstinent subjects. Plasma
luteinizing hormone levels were significantly lower (p<0.01)
in the heroin using subjects than in the control and abstinent individuals. Eight of the 17 heroin users had plasma
LH levels which were in the subnormal range.

It was not possible to establish any correlation between
the reported frequency and dose of heroin used (as expressed
in Hong Kong dollar costs per unit dose) and the degree of
suppression of luteinizing hormone or testosterone. This was
presumably due to a rather wide variation in actual dose size
of heroin in equivalent cost packages procured on the illicit
drug market. However, there was a relatively good correlation
(r=.84) between degree of suppression of luteinizing hormone
and suppression of testosterone observed in the active heroin
users.

DUSCUSSION

A significant suppression of luteinizing hormone and testosterone levels in active heroin users is consistent with well
documented effects of acute opiate administration in both experimental animals and humans (2). These data are also consistent with findings obtained in previous studies of active
heroin users in Hong Kong (7). Although heroin (alone and in
combination with methadone) significantly suppressed testosterone levels in adults (mean age=30), testosterone levels
returned to normal after about 1 month of abstinence from
opiates (7).
Chronic heroin use during puberty did not appear to ad-
versely affect psychosexual growth and development, even in
a young man who began heroin use during early puberty, at age
11. These data are inconsistent with our previous observation
of abnormally low plasma testosterone levels (118 mcg/100 ml)
in a 15 year old boy, abstinent from heroin for 3 months, who
had begun using it at age 12 (7).
Normal psychosexual growth and development observed in 16
subjects who began heroin use during puberty suggests that
despite recurrent heroin-induced suppression of pituitary gonadal hormones, adaptive or compensatory mechanisms occur and
pubertal development is not disrupted. This adaptive process
is probably due in part to feedback control of steroids on
gonadotrophin secretory activity. When opioid drugs suppress
LH, the subsequent decrement in plasma testosterone stimulates
enhanced production of LH which, in part, overrides the initial suppressive effects of the drug on LH secretion.
Interpretation of these data are limited by the fact that
it was impossible to accurately reconstruct dose-time patterns
of heroin self-administration by the active heroin users and
the abstinent subjects. It is reasonable to assume that heroin
doses taken by inhalation of pyrolized pure heroin were high.
However, it is difficult to equate inhalation and intravenous
administration. The possibility that more frequent and sus-

tained self-administration of heroin via an intravenous route
would produce greater impairment of pituitary gonadal hormones and psychosexual development cannot be excluded on the
basis of these findings.

ACKNOWLEDGEMENTS

   This research was supported in part by Grants DA 4 RG 010,
DA 016-76, DA 02905 and KO5 DA 00064 from the National Institute on Drug Abuse, ADAMHA. We are grateful to Mr. James M.N.
Ch'ien and the staff of the Society for the Aid and Rehabilitation of Drug Addicts (SARDA), Hong Kong, whose generous
assistance made these studies possible. We also thank Sir
Albert Rodrigues, Dr. J.B. Hollinrake, and Mr. Anthony Choy
for their contributions to these studies. Finally, we are
grateful to the staff of the American Consulate, Hong Kong,
who provided essential support and assistance for this research.

REFERENCES

1. Azizi, F., Vagenakis, A., Longcope, C., Ingbar, S.H. and
       Braverman, L.E. (1973). *Steroids* <u>22</u>, 467-472.
2. Cicero, T.J. (1980). *In* "Advances in Substance Abuse, Be-
       havioral and Biological Research" (Ed. N.K. Mello).
       Vol. 1, pp. 201-254. JAI Press, Inc., Greenwich, Conn.
3. Cicero, T.J., Bell, R.D., Wiest, R.G., Allison, J.H.,
       Polakoski, K. and Robins, E. (1975). *New Eng. J. Med.*
       <u>292</u>, 882-887.
4. Grumbach, M.M. (1980). *In* "Neuroendocrinology" (Eds D.T.
       Krieger and J.C. Hughes). pp. 249-258. H.P. Publishing
       Co., New York.
5. Martin, W.R., Jasinski, D.R., Haertzen, C.A., Kay, D.C.,
       Jones, B.E., Mansky, P.A. and Carpenter, R.W. (1973).
       Arch. Gen. Psychiatry <u>28</u>, 286-295.
6. Mendelson, J.H. and Mello, N.K. (1974). *In* "Aggression"
       (Ed. S.H. Frazier). pp. 225-247. Williams and Wilkins
       Co., Baltimore.
7. Mendelson, J.H. and Mello, N.K. (1975). *Clin. Pharmacol.*
       Ther. <u>17</u>, 529-533.
8. Mendelson, J.H., Mello, N.K. and Ellingboe, J. (1977).
       J. Pharmac. Exp. Ther. <u>202</u>, 676-682.
9. Mendelson, J.H., Mendelson, J.E. and Patch, V.D. (1975).
       J. Pharmac. Exp. Ther. <u>192</u>, 211-217.
10. Mendelson, J.H., Ellingboe, J., Kuehnle, J.C. and Mello,
       N.K. (1980). *J. Pharmacol. Exp. Ther.* <u>214</u>, 503-506.

11. Mendelson, J.H., Ellingboe, J., Mello, N.K. and Kuehnle, J.C. (1978). *Alcoholism: Clin. Exp. Res.* 2, 255-258.
12. Mendelson, J.H., Kuehnle, J.C., Ellingboe, J. and Babor, T.F. (1974). *New Eng. J. Med.* 291, 1051-1055.
13. Mendelson, J.H., Kuehnle, J.C., Ellingboe, J. and Babor, T.F. (1975). *In* "Marihuana and Health Hazards: Methodological Issues in Current Research" (Ed. J. Tinklenberg). pp. 83-93. Academic Press, New York.
14. Mendelson, J.H., Meyer, R.E., Ellingboe, J., Mirin, S.M., and McDougle, M. (1975). *J. Pharmac. Exp. Ther.* 195, 296-302.
15. Midgley, A.R. (1966). *Endocrinology* 79, 10-18.
16. Mirin, S.M., Meyer, R.E., Mendelson, J.H. and Ellingboe, J. (1980). *Amer. J. Psychiatry* 137, 909-915.
17. Niswender, G.D., Reichert, L.E., Midgley, A.R. and Nalbandov, A.C. (1969). *Endocrinology* 84, 1166-1173.
18. Rubin, H.B. and Henson, D.E. (1976). *Psychopharmacologia* 47, 123-134.
19. Wieland, W.E. and Younger, M. (1970). *In* "Proceedings of the Third National Conference on Methadone Treatment" pp. 50-53. U.S. Government Printing Office, Washington, D.C.
20. Wilson, G.T. (1981). *In* "Advances in Substance Abuse, Behavioral and Biological Research" (Ed. N.K. Mello) Vol. 2, pp. 1-40, JAI Press, Inc., Greenwich, Conn.

Portions of this paper were originally published in *Neurobehavioral Toxicology and Teratology* and are reproduced with permission of the publisher.

OPIATE INVOLVEMENT IN PROLACTIN AND GROWTH HORMONE
RELEASE IN MAN

George Tolis*(+) and Angelos Yotis+

*McGill University, Montreal, Canada

+Division of Endocrinology
Hippokrateion Hospital, 115 27, Athens, Greece

INTRODUCTION

Endogenous opioid peptides (EOP) modulate physiological, behavioral and endocrine parameters. These effects are due to specific interactions with different classes of opioid receptors designated as μ, κ, δ, ∂, ε, which are distributed in neuroactive sites both at C.N.S. and peripheral regions. Immunohistochemical studies have identified enkephalin, beta-endorphin and dynorphin-like opioid peptides to represent three major systems of EOP. The role of these peptides in the regulation of neurovegetative functions is still under intensive investigation.

This paper deals with the role of EOP and also exogenously administered opiates and antagonists on the release of growth hormone (GH) and prolactin (PRL) in man. An exaustive review of the pertinent literature covering the last five years is included. Yet, it should be pointed out that extrapolations of the involvement of EOP in the regulation of endocrine functions can only be made for specific protocols and by no means rule in or out the participation of such peptides in neuroendocrine mechanisms.

The studies to be reported are based either on acutely administered opioid receptor agonists or on the modifications of basal and stimulated GH and PRL release effected by Naloxone (Tables 1-5).

DOPAMINE AND NEUROENDOCRINE   Copyright© 1985 by Academic Press Inc. (London) Ltd.
ACTIVE SUBSTANCES   All rights of reproduction in any form reserved
ISBN 0 12 209045 4

EFFECT OF OPIOID RECEPTOR AGONISTS ON PRL AND GH

Prolactin

   Early studies in human subjects (1) revealed that morphine
raised serum PRL significantly with peak levels attained after
45 min. This profile resembled the dopamine-receptor blocking
agents rather than TRH and led to the hypothesis that opiates
may stimulate PRL release via an anti-dopaminergic mechanism.
Subsequent studies by the same group (2) indicated that dopaminomimetic drugs such as levodopa, apomorphine and bromocriptine at low single doses effectively prevented morphine-in-
duced PRL rise, whereas the anti-serotoninergic drug cyproheptadine at full doses was ineffective in doing so. In these early
acute studies no changes in plasma levels of GH, TSH, FSH, LH
and cortisol were recorded. However, the administration of
morphine to menopausal women elicited not only a rise in plasma
PRL, but also a substantial reduction in LH levels (3). This
effect has also been recently reported in male subjects (4).
In order to evaluate whether the PRL response to morphine and
subsequently to methadone took place via a specific interaction
with opiate receptors, we investigated whether naloxone at
low doses could prevent or blunt the stimulatory effects of
morphine on PRL release: our data confirmed this effect (1,2).
Similar results were reported for morphine and methadone (4),
although in these investigations high doses of naloxone were
used (Table 1); whether such high doses of naloxone operate
only via EOP receptor modification remains to be demonstrated.
   Subsequent to the discovery of EOP and knowing in the PRL-
stimulatory effect of morphine, a number of investigators have
searched for a PRL-secretagogue activity of endorphins and
enkephalins. Thus, administration of β-endorphin intravenously or intrathecally to healthy volunteers, drug addicts, depressed subjects and patients with pain due to disseminated
cancer resulted in an increase in serum PRL (6-10) (Table 2).
Although this finding is of interest, it could be predicted
from previous animal and human studies. There were, however,
some non endocrine findings that made the previous studies
worthwhile. For example, in the depression study a dissoci-
ation was detected between the decrease in heart-rate and the
depression of respiratory function induced by morphine. Since
this opiate as well as β-endorphin stimulated PRL secretion,
the existence of various receptor subtypes can be assumed,
whose activation is probably both dose and drug dependent.
The simultaneous study of a series of hormonal parameters
during infusion of different opiate receptor agonists supports

TABLE 1

Neuroendocrinology of opiate peptides
Effects on prolactin (1)

SUBSTANCE	DOSE	ROUTE	SUBJECTS	FINDINGS	REF.
Morphine	5-10 mg	i.v.	Scheduled for surg.	Rise	1
Morphine	5 mg	i.v.	Menopause	Rise	3
Morphine	10 mg	i.v.	Normal	Rise	4
Morphine plus Levodopa or Apomorph or Bromocrp	5-10 mg 500 mg 0.75 mg 2.5 mg	i.v. p.o. s.c. p.o.	Normal	Partial Blockade of PRL rise induced by Morph.	2
Morphine plus Naloxone Morphine plus Naloxone	5-10 mg 0.8 mg 10 mg 4 mg	i.v. i.v. i.v. i.v.	Normal	Blockade of PRL rise induced by Morph.	5
Methadone	40-60 mg	p.o.	Withdr. Addicts	Rise	2
Methadone	10 mg	i.v.	Normal	Rise	4
Methadone plus Levodopa or Apomorph or Bromocrp	500 mg 0.75 mg 2.5 mg	p.o. s.c. p.o.	Addicts on de- toxifica- tion	Partial Blockade	2
Methadone plus Naloxone	10 mg 4 mg	i.v. i.v.	Normal	Blockade	4

such a contention (4). Among the endorphins, specificity as a
PRL inhibitor seems indicative of the β-one, since experiments
conducted with a γ-endorphin analogue led to the opposite
effect (10).

  Although the precise mechanism of PRL release by morphine,
methadone and the untriacontapeptide β-endorphin is not fully
understood, the current belief is that these substances de-

TABLE 2

Neuroendocrinology of opiate peptides
Effects on prolactin (2)

SUBSTANCE	DOSE	ROUTE	SUBJECTS	FINDINGS	REF.
β-Endorphin	2.5 mg	i.v.	Normal	Rise	6
β-Endorphin	4.3-15 mg	i.v.	Depressed, withdrawing addicts	Rise	7
β-Endorphin	3 mg	intra-thecal	Patients with pain due to cancer	Rise	8
β-Endorphin plus Arginine	2.5 mg 500mg/kg	i.v.	Normal	Further rise in-duced by β-Endor	9
Des-Tyr-γ-Endorphin	1mg/day/ 10 days	i.m.	Schizo-phrenics off meds for 3 weeks	Decrease	10
Dermorphin plus Naloxone	5.5. g/kg/ min x 30min 4 mg ↓ 1mg/kg/ min x 3 h.	i.v. i.v. bolus ↓ infu-sion	Normal	Increase then Blockade	11
Damme	0.5 mg	i.m.	Normal	Rise	12
Damme plus Naloxone	0.5 mg 4 mg	i.m. i.v.	Normal	Blockade	12
Damme	0.25 mg	i.v.	Normal	Rise	4
Damme plus Naloxone	0.25 mg 4 mg	i.v. i.v.	Normal	Blockade	4
Damme	0.25 mg	i.v.	Acromegal.	Rise	15

crease dopamine-firing from neurons originating in the tubero-infundibular system, thus removing the dopaminergic inhibition of the anterior pituitary lactotropes.

The recently discovered heptapeptides, designated as dermor-phins because of their presence in the skin of South American frogs also stimulate PRL release via a mechanism most likely involving hypothalamic opiate receptors (11). It is of interest

TABLE 3

Neuroendocrinology of opiate peptides
Effects on growth hormone (1)

SUBSTANCE	DOSE	ROUTE	SUBJECTS	FINDINGS	REF.
Morphine	5-10 mg	i.v.	Scheduled for elective surg.	No change	1
Morphine	10 mg	i.v.	Normal	No change	4
Methadone	40-60 mg	p.o.	Withdraw. Methadone addicts	No change	1
Methadone	10 mg	i.v.	Normal	Increase	4
Methadone plus Naloxone	10 mg 4 mg	i.v. i.v.	Normal	Blockade	4
β-Endorphin	2.5 mg	i.v.	Normal	No change	6
β-Endorphin	4.3-15 mg	i.v.	Depressed, withdr.Methad.addicts	No change	7
β-Endorphin	3 mg	intrathecal	Patients with pain due to canc.	No change	8

that dermorphin shares structural similarity to the met-enke-
phalin analogue FK 33-824 or Damme, and similar to it, but
unlike morphine or β-endorphin, stimulates PRL and GH release. Dermorphin-like immunoreactivity has also been found
in methanol extracts of amphibian and rat brain. The met-
enkephalin analogue DAMME (D-ala^2-Mephe^4-met(O)-ol, FK 33-824)
has been shown to stimulate the release of PRL, GH and TSH
and to decrease ACTH and LH release (4,12-14), and it is
thought to activate both μ and δ receptor sites.

The precise mechanism of PRL release after the administration of exogenous and endogenous ligands to opiate receptors
is still obscure, but the ability of all of the different
kinds of opiate-receptor modulators to raise PRL is uncertain;
the teleology of the phenomenon is , however, as yet unknown.
The reports on PRL-release in some disease states (15) are
simply descriptive and not informative.

TABLE 4

Neuroendocrinology of opiate peptides
Effects on growth hormone (2)

SUBSTANCE	DOSE	ROUTE	SUBJECTS	FINDINGS	REF.
β-Endorphin plus	2.5 mg	i.v.	Normal	Blockade of Argin- ine induc. rise	9
Arginine	500 mg	i.v.			
Des-Tyr-γ Endorphin	1mg/day for 10 days	i.m.	Schizo- phrenics off meds for 3 wks	No change	10
Dermorphin	5.5µg/kg/ min x 30 min	i.v.	Normal	Increase	27
Dermorphin plus Naloxone	5.5·µg/kg/ min x 30 min ↓ 4 mg ↓ 1µg/kg/min for 3 hours	i.v. i.v. bol. ↓ i.v. inf.	Normal	Partial Blockade	27
Damme	0.5 mg	i.m.	Normal	Rise	12
Damme plus Naloxone	4 mg	i.v.	Normal	Blockade	12
Damme	0.25 mg	i.v.	Normal	Rise	4
Damme plus Naloxone	4 mg	i.v.	Normal	Blockade	4
Damme	0.25 mg	i.v.	Acromeg.	No change	15

Growth Hormone

Most of the studies employing morphine, methadone or β-endorphin fail to show that there is a GH stimulatory effect of these substances (Table 3,4). In contrast, both dermorphin and DAMME are capable of doing so (Table 4). As mentioned earlier, these differential effects of opioid receptor agonists upon GH and PRL release strongly suggest different types of receptors involved in the neuroendocrine effects of these drugs (4).

It should be pointed out that the same peptides which are unable to stimulate a hormone (i.e. β-endorphin on GH) may alter GH output if administered under certain conditions; β-

TABLE 5

Naloxone effects on GH and PRL dynamics in man

	PROLACTIN	GROWTH HORMONE	REFERENCE
BASAL			
Normal subjects	Nil	Nil	25,26
Puerperal women	Nil		20,21
Patients with			
– Acromegaly	Nil	Nil	15,24
– Prolactinoma	Nil	Nil	24
BREAST STIMULATION	Nil		20
SLEEP RELATED INCREASE	Nil	Nil	18,19
EXERCISE INDUCED RISE	Antagonizes	Antagonizes	16
FOOD INGESTION	Nil		17
OPIATE INDUCED RISE			
– Morphine	Blocks		1–4
– Methadone	Blocks	Blocks	2,4
– β-Endorphin	Blocks		6
– Dermorphin	Blocks	Blocks	11,27
– Damme	Blocks	Blocks	4,12
HYPOGLYCEMIA	Nil	Nil	28
TRH	Nil		26
CATECHOLAMINE ACTIVE DRUGS			
– Metoclopramide	Nil		29
– Apomorphine	Nil	Nil	30
– Clonidine		Nil	31
COLD PRESSOR TEST	Nil	Nil	22
ELECTROACUPUNCTURE			
– Normal subjects		Nil	23
– Patients with pain		Blocks	23

endorphin, for example, which does not stimulate GH release
per se, augments the stimulatory effect of arginine (9) and
can also decrease GH release under certain conditions (8).
    Thus, any substance which activates opiate receptors in
critical neuroendocrine areas may or may not always elicit
the same response; this depends on the dose, route of adminis-

tration and experimental protocols. The universal stimulatory
effects of all opiergic receptor activators upon prolactin
and their selective action upon GH, TSH, ACTH, LH/FSH is un-
doubtedly of great interest and calls for refined protocols
to unravel the significance of these observations.

EFFECT OF NALOXONE UPON PRL AND GH SECRETION

    In an effort to further delineate the specificity of the
results obtained with opiate substances on GH and PRL secretion, studies were carried out whereby the specific opiate receptor blocker naloxone was given. The work could be divided
into that assessing the effect of naloxone on PRL and GH release observed under basal conditions and/or physiologically
occurring situations e.g. sleep and that assessing whether
naloxone can modify the hormonal effect of opioid receptor
stimulants (Table 5). The available data up to now show no
evidence that naloxone at various doses can modify basal GH
or PRL secretion. Furthermore, with the exception of its possible inhibitory effect upon exercise induced GH or PRL rise
(16), there is nothing to suggest that it alters lactogen release induced by food ingestion (17) sleep (18,19), *puerperium*
or breast feeding (20,21). On the other hand it is very effective in minimizing or preventing the effects of opiergic substances upon both PRL and GH release (Tables 1-5).
    In contrast, when non-opiergic PRL and GH stimulants are
used, naloxone has no effect on either response pattern (Table 5); this strongly suggests that these agents i.e. apomorphine, clonidine, metoclopramide and TRH as well as insulin
induced hypoglycemia do not operate via endogenous opiate receptors. Thus, hypoglycemia has been used as a stressor to
affect anterior pituitary hormone release. Yet, the inability
of naloxone to block its action as well as that of the cold
pressor test upon PRL and GH release (22) questions the hypothesis that endogenous opiates play a role in stress or pain
related GH/PRL release. As a matter of fact, the observation
that electroacupuncture, which produced *analgesia* in chronic
pain patients, stimulates GH but not PRL release (23) contrasts
to previous contentions and, furthermore, points to the complexity of the issue.
    Up to now there has been no data to suggest a use for nalo-
xone in conditions whereby PRL and GH secretion is augmented
(15,24), nor has there been concrete evidence that its use can
delineate physiopathological mechanisms related to these hormones.

REFERENCES

1. Tolis, G., Hickey, T. and Guyda, H. (1975). *J. Clin. Endocrinol. Metab.* 41, 797-800.
2. Tolis, G., Dent, R. and Guyda, H. (1978). *J. Clin. Endocrinol. Metab.* 47, 200-203.
3. Hemmings, R., Fox, G. and Tolis, G. (1982). *Fertil. Steril.* 37, 389-391.
4. Delitala, G., Grossman, A. and Besser, M. (1983). *Neuroendocrinology* 37, 275-279.
5. Tolis, G., Ruggere, D., Pinter, E. and Panovac, K. (1978). *Endocrinology* 102, 359.
6. Reid, R.L., Hoff, J.D., Yen, S.S. and Li, C.H. (1981). *J. Clin. Endocrinol. Metab.* 52, 1179-1184.
7. Catlin, D.H., Gorelick, D.A., Gerner, R.H., Hui, K.K. and Li, C.H. (1980). *Arch. Gen. Psychiatry* 37, 635-640.
8. Oyama, T., Yamaya, R., Jin, T. and Kudo, T. (1982). *Acta Endocrinol. (Kbh)* 99, 9-13.
9. Reid, R.L. and Yen, S.S. (1981). *Life Sci.* 29, 2641-2647.
10. Verhoeven, W.M., Westenberg, H.G., Gerritsen, T.W., van Praag, H.M., Thijssen, J.H., Schwarz, F., van Ree, J.M. and de Wied, D. (1981). *Psychiatry Res.* 5, 293-309.
11. degli Uberti, E.C., Trasforini, G., Salvadori, S., Tomatis, R., Margutti, A., Bianconi, M., Rotola, C. and Pansini, R. (1983). *J. Clin. Endocrinol. Metab.* 56, 1032-1034.
12. del Pozo, E., von Graffenried, B., Brownell, J., Derrer, F. and Marbach, P. (1980). *Horm. Res.* 13, 90-97.
13. del Pozo, E., Martin-Perez, J., Stadelmann, A., Girard, J. and Brownell, J. (1980). *J. Clin. Invest.* 65, 1531-1534.
14. del Pozo, E. and Köbberling, J. (1981). *In* "Research on Fertility and Sterility" (Eds J. Cortés-Prieto, A. Campos da Paz and M. Neves-e-Castro), pp. 205-209. MTP Press Ltd., Lancaster (England).
15. Delitala, G., Giusti, M., Borsi, L., Devilla, L., Mazzochi, G., Lotti, G. and Giordano, G. (1981). *Horm. Res.* 15, 88-98.
16. Moretti, C., Fabbri, A., Gnessi, L., Cappa, M., Calzolari, A., Fraioli, F., Grossman, A. and Besser, G.M. (1983). *Clin. Endocrinol. (Oxf)* 18, 135-138.
17. Ishizuka, B., Quigley, M.E. and Yen, S.S. (1983). *J. Clin. Endocrinol. Metab.* 57, 1111-1116.
18. Martin, J.B., Tolis, G., Wood, I. and Guyda, H. (1979). *Brain Res.* 168, 210-213.
19. Delitala, G., Giusti, M., Rodriguez, G., Mazzochi, G.

Ferrini, S., Baccelliere, L., Montano, C., Rosadini, G. and Giordano, G. (1982). *Acta Endocrinol. (Kbh)* <u>100</u>, 321-326.

20. Lodico, G., Stoppelli, I., Delitala, G. and Maioli, M. (1983). *Fertil. Steril.* <u>40</u>, 600-603.

21. Grossman, A., West, S., Williams, J., Evans, J., Rees, L.H. and Besser, G.M. (1982). *Clin. Endocrinol. (Oxf)* <u>16</u>, 317-320.

22. Volaka, J., Baumann, J., Pevnick, J., Reker, D., James, B. and Cho, D. (1980). *Psychoneuroendocrinology* <u>5</u>, 225-234.

23. Pullan, P.T., Finch, P.M., Yuen, R.W. and Watson, F.E. (1983). *Life Sci.* <u>32</u>, 1705-1709.

24. Tolis, G., Jukier, L., Wiesen, M., Krieger, D.T. (1982). *J. Clin. Endocrinol. Metab.* <u>54</u>, 780-784.

25. Naber, D., Pickar, D., Davis, G.C., Cohen, R.M., Jimerson, D.C., Elchisak, M.A., Defraites, E.G., Kalin, N.H. Risch, S.C. and Buchsbaum, M.S. (1981). *Psychopharmacology (Berlin)* <u>74</u>, 125-128.

26. Rolandi, E., Marabini, A., Magnani, G., Sannia, A. and Barreca, T. (1982). *Eur. J. Clin. Pharmacol.* <u>22</u>, 213-216.

27. degli Uberti, E.C., Trasforini, G., Salvadori, S., Margutti, A., Tomatis, R., Rotola, C., Bianconi, M. and Pansini, R. (1983). *Neuroendocrinology* <u>37</u>, 280-283.

28. Wakabayashi, I., Demura, R., Miki, N., Ohmura, E., Miyoshi, H. and Shizume, K. (1980). *J. Clin. Endocrinol. Metab.* <u>50</u>, 597-599.

29. Delitala, G., Devilla, L. and Musso, N.R. (1983). *J. Clin. Endocrinol. Metab.* <u>56</u>, 181-184.

30. Rowbotham, M.C., Joseph, M.S., Jones, R.T. and Keil, L.C. (1983). *Psychoneuroendocrinology* <u>8</u>, 95-102.

31. Massara, F., Limone, P., Cagliero, E., Tagliabue, M., Isaia, G.C. and Molinatti, G.M. (1983). *Acta Endocrinol. (Kbh)* <u>103</u>, 371-375.

STIMULATION-ASSOCIATED RELEASE OF ENDORPHINS

Fred Nyberg, Anders Neil and Lars Terenius

*Department of Pharmacology, Uppsala University,
Biomedical Center, Box 573, S-751 23 Uppsala, Sweden*

Associations between painful stimulation or stressful conditions and the release of endorphins have been studied extensively during the last decade. These morphine-like peptides and their receptors have been localized in many areas of the central nervous system (CNS) and are potentially important in central control and modulatory systems for pain.

The large family of opioid peptides appears to represent a very flexible and widespread signalling system. Recent work with cDNA technology and gene cloning has now revealed the existence of at least three genetically distinct opioid peptide precursors: proopiomelanocortin, proenkephalin and prodynorphin. The precursors contain several neurohormonal units and enzymatic processing may produce a number of active peptides of various structure. Each endorphin system has its unique distribution within the nervous system and in endocrine tissue. Furthermore, it has been possible, even with still relatively crude probes, to distinguish a minimum of at least three types of opioid receptors, mu, delta and kappa. In general, the peptides differ from classic opiate drugs in their receptor profile. Extrapolations from opiate pharmacology to endogenous systems may therefore be misleading.

CHEMICAL CHARACTERISTICS AND DISTRIBUTION OF OPIOID PEPTIDES

Following the identification of the enkephalin structures in 1975 (1) a variety of other endorphins have been isolated and sequenced (for review see ref. 2). A common structural unit of all these peptides is the N-terminus with the amino acid sequence Tyr–Gly–Gly–Phe. In the enkephalins there is C-terminal extension with a Met or Leu residue; in the other endorphins the sequences

TABLE 1

Structure of the opioid peptides

Precursor/Peptide	Structures
Proopiomelanocortin	
beta-endorphin	Tyr-Gly-Gly-Phe-Met-Thr-Ser-Glu-Lys-
	-Ser-Gln-Thr-Pro-Leu-Val-Thr-Leu-Phe-
	-Lys-Asn-Ala-Ile-Ile-Lys-Asn-Ala-Tyr-
	-Lys-Lys-Gly-Glu
alfa-endorphin	1-16 sequence
gamma-endorphin	1-17 sequence
delta-endorphin	1-27 sequence
Proenkephalin	
(Leu)enkephalin	Tyr-Gly-Gly-Phe-Leu
(Met)enkephalin	Tyr-Gly-Gly-Phe-Met
(Met)enkephalin-Lys^6	Tyr-Gly-Gly-Phe-Met-Lys
(Met)enkephalin-Arg$_6$-Phe$_7$	Tyr-Gly-Gly-Phe-Met-Arg-Phe
(Met)enkephalin-Arg^6-Gly^7-Leu^8	Tyr-Gly-Gly-Phe-Met-Arg-Gly-Leu
Prodynorphin	
Dynorphin A	Tyr-Gly-Gly-Phe-Leu-Arg-Arg-Ile-Arg-
	-Pro-Lys-Leu--Lys-Trp-Asp-Asn-Glu
Dynorphin A (1-8)	1-8 sequence
Dynorphin B	Tyr-Gly-Gly-Phe-Leu-Arg-Arg-Gln-
(Rimorphin)	-Phe-Lys-Val-Val-Thr
alfa-neoendorphin	Tyr-Gly-Gly-Phe-Leu-Arg-Lys-Tyr-Pro-
	-Lys
beta-neoendorphin	1-9 sequence

are elongated and peptides with as much as 30 amino acid residues have been isolated (Table 1). Processing of the proopiomelanocortin precursor (3) is known to generate beta-endorphin and fragments. Proenkephalin (4) contains within its structure six copies of (Met)enkephalin and one copy (Leu)enkephalin and may give rise to a variety of enkephalin – related peptides (Table 1). The prodynorphin precursor (5) contains the sequences of three unique (Leu)enkephalin peptides: alfa–neoendorphin, dynorphin A and dynorphin B. Other (Leu)enkephalin–containing peptides consisting of fragments or combinations of these three peptides have also been characterized (Table I).

As mentioned above, besides the chemical variety there is also a variety of tissues producing these peptides. Immunohistochemical mapping and radioimmuno-assay measurements suggest that the CNS distribution of beta-endorphin and dynorphin is different from that of the enkephalins (6,7,8). Enkephalins are ubiquitous and widely distributed within the CNS (including the spinal cord) whereas beta-endorphin-containing elements (besides the adenohypophysis) are present in limbic structures including the septal area, medial thalamus and midbrain periaqueductal grey down to the locus coeruleus. Dynorphin peptides occur in high concentrations in the neurohypo-physis, in the substantia nigra and hypothalamus and in lower concentrations in other brain nuclei and spinal areas (9).

OPIOID RECEPTORS

Current evidence indicates the existence of multiple types of opioid receptors (for review see ref. 10). On the basis of biochemical and pharmacological studies they have been subdivided into three main types: the mu, delta and kappa receptors. Each of these receptors has been characterized for its affinity for specific ligands. Whereas selective mu and delta ligands are available (e.g. dihydromorphine and Tyr-D-Thr-Gly-Phe-Leu-Thr, respectively), the kappa ligands (e.g. bremazocine or ethylketocyclazocine) display the common disadvantage of interaction with high affinity for all three receptors. Evidence for the existence of a fourth binding site perhaps corresponding to the sigma-receptor has also been reported (e.g. 11). In a recent study (Neil, manuscript in preparation) we were able to detect and characterize four binding sites in mouse brain membranes three of which may correspond to mu-, delta- and kappa receptors, respectively. The fourth site bound ethylketocyklazocine with comparatively high affinity, whereas the affinity for mu and delta ligands was negligible. Fig. 1 illustra-tes the relative affinities of various ligands towards the four different binding sites. Considering their high affinity for morphine the mu receptors are considered to be specially involved in analgesia and have been frequ-ently studied with pharmacological techniques. A common approach has been the use of receptor antagonists such as naloxone. This compound with high affinity for mu sites antagonizes the major analgesic actions of opiates and endorphins and has also been used to investigate other

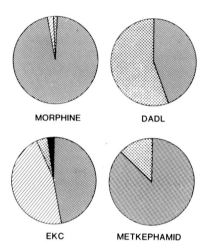

Fig. 1. *The relative affinities of morphine, D-Ala²-Leu⁵-enkephalin (DALE), ethylketocyclazocine (EKC) and metkemphamid towards four binding sites in the mouse brain. The sectors represent the association constants for a given site in percent of the sum of the affinity constants towards the four sites, where (∷) dotted sector represents mu, checked (⧣) is delta, striped (⫽) kappa and filled (■) the fourth site, respectively.*

physiological effects of endorphins. However, there is evidence that both kappa and delta receptors also can modulate nociception at the spinal cord level, and that they differ with regard to the noxious modalities they inhibit (12).

The receptor preference of endogenous opioids has also been the subject of extensive studies. It appears that e.g. the enkephalins are ligands for mu and delta receptors, whereas dynorphin and other C-terminally elongated (Leu)-enkephalins bind quite specifically to kappa receptors. The (Met)enkephalin extensions with Arg-Phe and Arg-Gly-Leu at the C-terminus have affinity for both delta and kappa sites.

OPIOID PEPTIDES AND PAIN

In recent years the relation between endorphins and pain modulation has been subjected to extensive studies (for review see ref. 13). The periaqueductal grey region in the brain stem has been found to have a key function partly via descending systems inhibiting pain transmission at the spinal level (14,15). The importance of spinal modulation goes back to the early gate-control theory (16), which postulated a modulation of nociceptive signals at the spinal level. Recent work on opioid peptides and opioid receptor distribution has reinforced the importance of the dorsal spinal cord in pain control.

Studies of endogenous opioids in relation to the mechanism of pain modulation have been performed in the context of two experimental paradigms: stress-induced analgesia and stimulation-produced analgesia (SPA). Stress-induced analgesia has been shown to involve both opioid and non-opioid components (17-19). Direct evidence for the activation of the beta-endorphin (20) and enkephalin (21) systems by stress has been reported.

An important link between the endorphins and analgesia has developed from the early observation (22) that electric stimulation of periaqueductal areas in rat brain produce surgical analgesia. This demonstration has now been proved by several studies of various design and involving a variety of species (23). SPA has also been shown to be partially reversed by naloxone (24). Moreover, evidence for the release of opioid peptides in central as well as in peripheral SPA has accumulated. In a recent study made in collaboration with Dr. J.-S. Han (Beijing Medical College, China) evidence for a causal relationship between endorphin release induced by acupuncture and analgesic response was observed (25). Thus, microinjection of (Met)enkephalin or beta-endorphin antibodies into periaqueductal grey matter of rabbits significantly reduced the analgesia obtained by electroacupuncture. However, when the antibodies were injected intrathecally a reduction of the analgesia was only obtained by the (Met)enkephalin antibodies. This observation is consonant with the rich enkephalinergic innervation in spinal cord and the absence of beta-endorphin fibers.

Support for a pain inhibitory role of the opioid peptides has also emerged from pharmacological experiments with exogenous administration of endorphins. For instance, beta-endorphin has been shown to produce a potent and

long-lasting analgesic activity after intracerebroventri-
cular injection (26,27), whereas enkephalins when administered in a similar fashion were found to be weakly
analgesic (28). Central administration of dynorphin has
also been demonstrated to produce analgesia (29).

CHARACTERIZATION OF OPIOID PEPTIDES RELEASED DURING STIMULATION-PRODUCED ANALGESIA

Changes in the content and release of opioid peptides
during various type of stimulation has also been observed
in many laboratories. Selective brain stimulation leads
to analgesia and increased release of beta-endorphin in
the cerebrospinal fluid (CSF) (30). In this laboratory it
was shown that transcutaneous nerve stimulation (TNS) also
resulted in increase of opioid peptides in lumbar CSF
from patients with neurogenic pain (31). Electroacupuncture in heroin addicts has been found to raise CSF
(Met)enkephalin without altering plasma concentrations
(32). Noxious stimuli may also lead to incresed endorphin
release; thus an increase in spinal enkephalin levels has
been demonstrated in polyarthritic rats (33). Increased
levels of CSF (Met)enkephalin in cats have also been
detected after high intensity sciatic nerve stimulation
(34) and after stimulation of the tooth pulp (35).
A model for the study of the release of endorphins
in SPA has been established in collaboration with Dr. T.
Yaksh (Mayo Clinic, Rochester, USA) (36). Anesthetized
cats are prepared for spinal superfusion with a concentric
polyethylene catheter inserted through the cisternal
membrane. Artificial CSF with albumin and bacitracin is
infused through the inner catheter which extended to the
sacral cord. The outflow is collected through the outer
catheter which extended to the mid-thoracic cord. CSF-
material is collected before and during high intensity
stimulation of the sciatic nerve. The superfusates are
fractionated and analyzed by various biochemical techniques and the endorphin activity measured by radioimmuno-
and radioreceptorassays. From these experiments it became
clear that the CSF concentration of endogenous opioids
(as determined by radioreceptor assay) displayed a
significant increase during stimulation conditions.
However, over 70% of the released activity showed a
chromatographic behaviour, which was different from those
of beta-endorphin and enkephalins. Fractionation on
Sephadex G-10 yielded the receptor-active material into
two separate fractions eluting ahead of (FI) and later

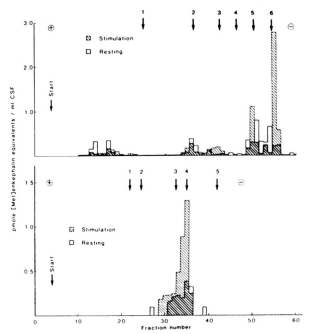

Fig. 2. The distribution of receptor activity after electro-phoresis in agarose suspension of the FI (upper panel) and FII (lower panel) material in spinal perfusate from anesthet-ized cats. Perfusion was carried out at resting condition and during high intensity bilateral stimulation of the sciatic nerves. Samples collected during resting and stimulation were run at 1000V for 6h in 0.1M ammonium formate, pH 2.7. The column was calibrated with (upper panel): 1 = (Leu)Enk; 2 = (Leu)Enk-Arg⁶; 3 = dynorphin (1-8); 4 = dynorphin; 5 = alfa-neoendorphin; 6 = dynorphin (1-13); (lower panel): 1 = (Met) Enk; 2 = (Leu)Enk; 3 = (Met)Enk-Arg⁶-Phe⁷; 4 = (Met)Enk-Lys⁶; 5 = dynorphin (1-8).

than (FII) the salt peak. Radioimmunoasssay indicated a significant increase of dynorphin during stimulation. This peptide, however, appeared to represent a minor component of FI. Electrophoresis of the receptor active material revealed two principal peaks elicited in FI and one in FII (Fig. 2). The electrophoretic mobility of the activity observed in FII suggested that the increase was due to (Met)enkephalin Lys⁶. Further support for an identity between the FII component and this enkephalyl hexapeptide was obtained by radioimmunoassay and HPLC (37). Furthermore, enzymatic degradation experi-

ments coupled to radioimmunoassay provided evidence for
the presence of enkephalin pentapeptide sequences in all
three released components. Thus, the FII component
contained mainly the (Met)enkephalin sequence, whereas
the material elicited in FI consisted of both (Leu)- and
(Met)enkephalin. Apparently both the enkephalin and
dynorphin systems are activated by this somatic stimulation. It is not clear, however, whether these components
are the primary products of release or products resulting
from degradation processes. To settle this question additional studies will be needed. For that purpose studies
including addition of peptidase inhibitors to the perfusion
fluid has been initiated and are in progress.

CONCLUSIONS

The complexity of the opioid peptides and their
receptors is such that it is unlikely that drugs can be
discovered that selectively would probe one peptide
system. For instance, proenkephalin may generate enkephalins which have delta-receptor preference but also
C-terminally elongated peptides with increasing kappa-
-receptor selectively and the recently discovered metor-
phamide (38) which is mu-selective. Even the present use
of naloxone to distinguish opioid versus non-opioid
mechanisms may represent an over-simplification. Naloxone
is an efficacous mu-antagonist, a relatively less active
kappa-antagonist and a poor delta-antagonist. It is
entirely possible that certain peptides of the endorphin
family would produce analgesic effects which are hard to
antagonize by naloxone. Another consideration making it
difficult to probe the endorphin systems with drugs is
their complex and partially overlapping anatomical
distribution.

The chemical approaches to the study of release of
opioid peptides have similar limitations. The pluripotency
of opioid peptide precursors can potentially lead to a
very large family of active peptides. Furthermore, there
is evidence that precursor processing is qualitatively
different in different tissues, maybe CNS areas. Consequently, chemical methods need to be flexible enough to
accomodate a variety of structural variations but also
specific enough to distinguish individual components.
There is no single technology available which has both
these characteristics. The combination of techniques we
have used as illustrated above represents an attempt to
deal with the complexity. As indicated, the results are

partly unexpected, peptides identified with these techniques
are not those conventionally thought of as being the true
mediators in endorphinergic synapses. Whether they have a true
function or merely represent the stable remnants of the syn-
aptic activity, needs further studies. Clearly, it is of central importance to define which opioid peptides are being released in the different systems.

AKNOWLEDGEMENTS

These studies were supported by the Swedidh Medical Research Council and the National Institute on Drug Abuse,
Washington, D.C.

REFERENCES

1. Hughes, J., Smith, T.W., Kosterlitz, H.W. *et al.* (1975).
      Nature 258, 577-579.
2. Morley, J.S. (1983). *Br. Med. Bull.* 39, 5-10.
3. Nakanishi, S., Inoue, A., Kita, I. *et al.* (1979). *Nature*
      278, 423-427.
4. Gubler, U., Seeburg, P., Hoffman, B.J. *et al.* (1982).
      Nature 295, 206-208.
5. Kakidani, H., Furutani, Y., Takahashi, H. *et al.* (1982).
      Nature 298, 245-249.
6. Bloom, F.E., Rossier, J., Battenberg, E.L.F. *et al.* (1978).
      Adv. Biochem. Pharmacol. 18, 89-109.
7. Watson, S.J., Akil, H., Ghazarossian, V.E. *et al.* (1981).
      Proc. Natl. Acad. Sci. (USA) 78, 1260-1263.
8. Watson, S.J., Akil, H., Fischli, W. *et al.* (1982). *Science*
      216, 85-87.
9. Hertz, A., Hölt, V., Gramsch, C. *et al.* (1982). *In*
      "Regulatory Peptides: From Molecular Biology to
      Function" (Eds E. Costa and M. Trabucchi),pp. 55-59.
      Raven Press, New York.
10. Kosterlitz, H.W., Paterson, S.J., Robson, L.E. (1982).
      In "Neuropeptides: Basic and Clinical Aspects" (Eds
      G. Flink and L.J. Whalley). pp. 3-11, Churchill
      Livingstone, Edinburgh.
11. Sadée, W., Richards, M.L., Grevel, J. *et al.* (1983).
      Life Sci. 33, Suppl. 1, 187-189.
12. Yaksh, T.L. (1983). *J. Pharm. Exptl. Ther.* 226, 303-306.
13. Terenius, L. (1981). *Front. Horm. Res.* 8, 162-177.
14. Jacquet, Y.F. and Lajtha, A. (1974). *Science* 185, 1055-
      1057.
15. Yaksh, T.L. and Rudy, T.A. (1978). *Pain* 4, 299-359.

16. Melzack, R. and Wall, P.D. (1965). *Science* 150, 971-979.
17. Bodnar, R., Kelly, D., Spiagga, A. *et al.* (1978).
    Pharmacol. Biochem. Behav. 8, 667-672.
18. Lewis, J.W., Canon, J., Liebeskind, J. (1980). *Science*
    208, 623-625.
19. Lewis, J.W., Stapleton, J.M., Castiglioni, A.J. *et al.*
    (1982). *In* "Neuropeptides: Basic and Clinical Aspects"
    (Eds G. Flink and L.J. Whalley). pp. 41-49, Churchill
    Livingstone, Edinburgh.
20. Rossier, J., French, E.D., Rivier, C. *et al.* (1977).
    Nature 270, 618-620.
21. Stern, A.S., Lewis, R.V., Komura, S. *et al.* (1979).
    Proc. Natl. Acad. Sci. (USA) 76, 6680-6683.
22. Reynolds, D.V. (1969). *Science* 164, 444-445.
23. Han, J.S. and Terenius, L. (1982). *Ann. Rev. Pharmacol.*
    Toxicol. 22, 193-220.
24. Akil, H., Mayer, D. and Liebeskind, J. (1976). *Science*
    191, 961-962.
25. Han, J.S., Xie, G-X., Zhou, Z.-F. *et al.* (1982). *In*
    "Regulatory Peptides: From Molecular Biology to
    Function" (Eds E. Costa and M. Trabucchi). pp. 369-
    377, Raven Press, New York.
26. Loh, H.H., Tseng, L.F., Wei, E. *et al.* (1976). *Proc.*
    Natl. Acad. Sci. (USA) 73, 2895-2898.
27. Gráf, L., Szekaly, J.I., Rónai, A.Z. *et al.* (1976). *Nature*
    263, 240-242.
28. Belluzzi, J.D., Grant, N., Garsky, V. *et al.* (1976).
    Nature 260, 625-626.
29. Goldstein, A., Tachibana, S., Lownay, L. *et al.* (1979).
    Proc. Natl. Acad. Sci. (USA) 76, 6666-6670.
30. Akil, H., Richardson, D., Barchas, J. (1978). *Proc. Natl.*
    Acad. Sci. (USA) 7, 5170-5172.
31. Sjölund, B., Terenius, L. and Eriksson, M. (1977).
    Acta Physiol. Scand. 100, 382-384.
32. Clement-Jones, V., Lowry, P.J., McLoughlin, L. *et al.*
    (1979). *Lancet*, ii, 380-383,
33. Cesselin, F., Montastruc, J.L., Gros, C. *et al.* (1980).
    Brain Res. 191, 289-293.
34. Yaksh, T.L. and Elde, R.P. (1980). *Eur. J. Pharmacol.*
    63, 359-362.
35. Cesselin, F., Oliveras, J.L., Bourgoin, S. *et al.* (1982).
    Brain Res. 237, 325-338.
36. Yaksh, T.L., Terenius, L., Nyberg, F. *et al.* (1983). *Brain*
    Res. 268, 119-128.
37. Nyberg, F., Yaksh, T.L., Terenius, L. (1983). *Life Sci.* 33,
    suppl. 1, 17-20.
38. Weber, E., Esch, F.S., Böhlen, P. *et al.* (1983). *Proc.*
    Natl. Acad. Sci. (USA) 75, 5170-5172.

VI. Advances in Brain Peptide Research

PRE-AND POST-SECRETIONAL PROCESSING OF PRO-OPIOCORTIN

P.J. Lowry

Protein Hormone Unit, St. Bartholomew's Centre for Clinical Research, London EC1A 7BE, England.

PRO-OPIOCORTIN AND THE PARS INTERMEDIA

The structure of pro-opiocortin is infered from the sequence of complementary DNA synthesised on m-RNA template
extracted from the pars intermedia of bovine hypophyses (1).
It is a poly-peptide of some 240 residues (there are small
variations in this number between species) with ACTH occupying a central position and β-LPH and the C-terminal region. A cryptic melanotropin sequence is found in the middle of the remaining N-terminal section. As α and β-MSH are
found within the structures of ACTH and β-LPH respectively
this third melanotropic sequence is called γ-MSH (Fig.1).
Immunostaining the pars intermedia with a variety of antisera generated against different regions of pro-opiocortin
inevitably stains all the parenchymal cells of the pars
intermedia and constitute the bulk of this tissue (2). Pre-
secretional processing of the ACTH/LPH region of pro-opiocortin proceeds rapidly giving rise to a variety of small
peptides. In the rat α-MSH and CLIP are derived from the
ACTH region. C-terminally truncated, glycosylated and phos-
phorylated forms of CLIP are also found and α-MSH can occur
in the di or deacetylated forms (3-5) β-LPH is processed to
γ-LPH and β-endorphin is also acetylated. C-terminally
truncated forms of endorphin are also found which apparently
give rise to a   C-terminal dipeptide which can display
neurotransmitter properties (6). In other animals such as
pig and ox slight changes in the flanking dibasic residues
give rise to an extra processing site and β-MSH and N-terminal γ-LPH peptides rather than γ-LPH are the major peptides formed (7). The N-terminal peptide from pro-opiocortin (N-POC) containing the γ-MSH sequence quickly loses
a degenerate peptide from its C-terminus (this peptide

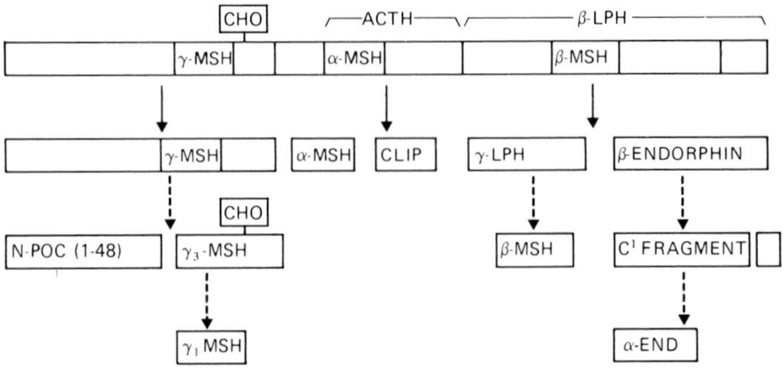

Fig. 1. The processing of pro-opiocortin in the mammalian pituitary. Vertical bars represent cleavage sites at dibasic residues. Pro-γ-MSH is N-POC (1-48) plus γ₃-MSH.

varies considerably in size and sequence between species) to give a large glycopeptide with γ_3-MSH occupying its C-terminus and has been called pro-γ-MSH. In the rat this peptide is 74 residues long and is one and the same as the 16K fragment originally described by Mains and Eipper (4). Although this peptide contains dibasic residues at positions 48/49 just in front of the γ_3-MSH sequence (N-POC (50-74)) cleavage at this position proceeds slowly for reasons which are not clear and only about 30% is processed to N-POC (1-48/49) and γ_3-MSH before secretion (4,8). Again because of changes in sequence a new dibasic residue cleavage site is found in the bovine sequence just after the γ-MSH sequence and this γ_3-MSH is further processed to two smaller peptides the one containing the γ-MSH losing its C-terminal glycine in the formation of a C-terminal amide (9). It is perhaps quite extraordinary that in spite of this plethora of information on the processing of what would appear in first glance, to be an enormous amount of potential biological information contained within these peptides, a true physiological role has yet to be ascribed to the pars intermedia in mammals. Even more surprising is the fact that all these peptides are secreted concomitantly from the pars intermedia under a common dopaminergic tonic inhibition mechanism (10) the tissue being directly innervated by dopaminergic neurones (11). The fact that several animals have little or no pars intermedia tissue at all (12) would suggest that the gland and its secreted peptides can be dispensed with. However the pars intermedia when it occurs does not give the impression of being vestigal as many of the peptides have been detected in the circulation (13). There have been sev-

eral reports ascribing biological activities to α-MSH such
as pigmentation, sebum secretion and its associated role in
the release of olfactory cues to promote aggresion, terri-
torial behaviour and sexual attraction; natriureses; lipolysis; pituitary hormone release (14); stimulation of foetal
body growth and brain development (15), in the initiation of
labour, and adrenal steroidogenic and growth promoting factor in the foetus (16,17) and in the release of aldosterone
from the rat zona glomerulosa (18). It is hard to imagine
that all these activities are associated with just one of
ten possible POC peptides released simultaneously from the pars
intermedia and is the basis of a subtle endocrine system of
which some animals do not even have the need! The human
pituitary has little pars intermedia cells in adult life although during foetal life a distinct zona intermedia can be
seen (12). Is it possible that in this case it is just another example of ontogeny recapturing phylogeny?

Post-secretional modification of pars intermedia peptides
has been described by Edwardson and his colleagues to be
caused by enzymes in the pars intermedia colloid which becomes particularly obvious after oestrogen treatment (19).
Indeed CLIP would appear to be processed to a smaller C-
terminal fragment before it can express insulin releasing
activity (20).

PRO-OPIOCORTIN AND THE PARS DISTALIS

Pro-opiocortin (POC) is also biosynthesised in the pars
distalis and like in the pars intermedia post translational
processing proceeds rapidly. In the case of the pars distalis the processing finishes at ACTH, β-LPH (with some 30%
γ-LPH and β-endorphin) and pro-γ-MSH((N-POC (1-76)) in the
human, and 1-74 in the rat). How the same precursor processing can finish so abruptly in the corticotropes of the pars
distalis when there are still dibasic residues (the signal
for processing) present within the structure of these molecules for their conversion into smaller pars intermedia-like
peptides is still unexplained. Simultaneous release of ACTH,
β-LPH (with some γ-LPH and β-endorphin), and pro-γ-MSH occurs
when the pars distalis is stimulated by the hypothalamus and
receives corticotropin releasing factors (CRF) in the
blood via the hypothalamic portal system. At least in this
case we have the well known and understood biological role
for ACTH, ie. stimulating steroidogenesis in the adrenal
cortex. Within seconds of an animal being stressed "CRF"
reaches the corticotropes of the pars distalis. No de novo
synthesis of ACTH or its cogeners are required as they

are stored in granules which can quickly secrete their contents on being stimulated. Recently, however, a potent CRF
isolated by Vale and his colleagues (21) has been shown to
increase pro-opiocortin m-RNA in the anterior pituitary (22).
The plasma ACTH concentration quickly rises within a few
minutes sufficiently to trigger the biosynthetic pathway
resulting finally in corticosteroidogenesis. This process
is slower than that required for ACTH release, taking several minutes as a labile protein has first to be synthesised
which transfers cholesterol into the mitochondrion. After
conversion to pregnenolone the enzymes required thereafter
are all constituitive and corticosteroidogenesis proceeds
rapidly(23). Until recently attempts to assign biological
roles to the other co-secreted pro-opiocortin peptides during
stress has proved elusive. Lipotropin peptides have been
proposed as having effects on lipolysis in fat cells (24)
and stimulating aldosterone secretion (25) but the doses
used in these studies was generally pharmacological and
there is little physiological basis for these claims. Although it is interesting to speculate that as β-endorphin
is formed from β-LPH the latter can act as a precursor for
opiate peptides, its concentration naturally being increased
during stress. Thus opiate peptides could be generated at
any injury site leading to local analgesia. There is not
however any evidence to this proposition. The N-terminal
region recently has proved to be a rich source of a variety
of peptides with interesting biological activities and has
dramatically increased our understanding of the control of
adrenal function. Pro-γ-MSH have been shown to potentiate
ACTH induced steroidogenesis (26,27) by activation of cholesterol ester hydrolyase (26) and by increasing RNA synthesis (28). Potentiation of steroidogenesis could also be
demonstrated with the trypsinised rat 16K fragment (N-POC
(1-74)) and with synthetic γ_3-MSH (29). We had been working
for many years on the hypothesis that adrenal growth and
hyperplasia were a consequence of a peptide being co-secreted with ACTH and had on realizing that it was β-LPH and not
"β-MSH" that was co-secreted with ACTH in humans (30,31)
we tested the adrenal growth promoting activity of β-LPH
only to find it inactive. Initially pro-γ-MSH also proved
to be inactive (32) but eventually it was found that smaller
peptides after being cleaved from the N-terminal region of
pro-γ-MSH were active both *in vivo* and *in vitro* in promoting
DNA synthesis and mitogenesis (33). As N-POC (1-74) is the
form secreted from the anterior pituitary of the rat under
the hypothalamic control of "CRF" we proposed that post
secretional cleavage of this peptide was the mechanism by

which adrenal growth and hyperplasia was controlled (23).
This hypothesis was corroborated by the observation that we
could inhibit certain aspects of compensatory growth of the remaining adrenal gland following unilateral adrenalectomy by
pretreating animals with various antisera directed against
regions of pro-γ-MSH. In particular an antiserum that had
been raised against the non-mitogenic end of N-POC (1-74)
ie. anti N-POC (50-74) or γ$_3$-MSH had the most dramatic effects of all inhibiting the increase in all three parameters
used to monitor compensatory adrenal growth (weight, RNA and
DNA) (34). As synthetic γ$_3$-MSH had been shown to be inactive in stimulating DNA synthesis *in vitro* (33) but its antiserum was inhibiting the expression of mitogenic activity
by binding to the pro-γ-MSH we reasoned that it must have
prevented cleavage thus inhibiting the latent activity. As
there was a wealth of information indicating that the control of compensatory adrenal growth was via a neural reflex
arc from one gland via the hypothalamus to the contralateral
gland, one gland   being able to grow independently of the
other (for review see 35) we concluded that the enzyme
which cleaved pro-γ-MSH which we now call the adrenal growth
factor (AGF) was found locally in the adrenal gland and was
somehow controlled by direct neural influences to release
the adrenal mitogenic hormone (N-POC (1-48/49) or AMH) and
the adrenal hypertrophic hormone (AHH, N-POC (50-74) or γ$_3$-
MSH) near or at the receptors on the adrenal cortical cells
(34). Thus the expression of biological activity of pro-γ-
MSH (AGF) can be controlled at two levels. Hypothalamic
"CRF" reaching the pituitary releases pro-γ-MSH along with
ACTH and potentiates their steroidogenic activity.
If one adrenal becomes damaged then a neural reflex activates a proteolytic enzyme in the contralateral gland releasing the mitogenic and hypertrophic hormones which stim-
ulate the gland to grow.

   This subtle control mechanism may not be restricted to
ACTH and its co-secreted cogeners, but the occurence of
other polyhormone precursors appear to be the rule rather
than the exception and neural activation of inactive precursors at specific target glands may prove to be a more
umbiquitous mechanism.

ACKNOWLEDGEMENTS

   The author wishes to thank Miss J.P. Bacon for her
typing of this review.

REFERENCES

1. Nakanishi, S., Inone, A., Kita, T., Nakamura, M., Chang,
    A.C.Y., Cohen, S.N. and Numa, S. (1979). *Nature* 278,
    423-427.
2. Kruseman, A.C.N. and Schroder-van de Elst, J.P. (1976).
    Virchows Arch. B. Cell Path. 22, 263-272.
3. Mains, R.E. and Eipper, B.A. (1981). *In* "Peptides of the
    Pars Intermedia". Ciba Foundation Symposium '81.
    Pitman Medical, London pp. 32-55.
4. Eipper, B.A. and Mains R.E. (1978). *J. Biol. Chem.* 253,
    5732-5744.
5. Browne, C.A., Bennett, H.P.J. and Solomon, S. (1981).
    Biochemistry 20, 4538-4546.
6. Parish, D.C., Smyth, D.G., Namanton, J.R.and Wolsten-
    croft, J.H. (1983). *Nature* 306, 267-270.
7. Hope, J. and Lowry, P.J. (1981). *Front. Horm. Res.* 8,
    44-61.
8. Jackson, S., Salacinski, P., Hope, J. and Lowry, P.J.
    (1983). *Peptides* 4, 431-438.
9. Bohlen, P., Esch, F., Shibasaki, T., Baird, A., Ling,
    N.and Guillemin, R. (1981). *Febs. Lett.* 128, 67-70.
10. Jackson, S. and Lowry, P.J. (1983). *Neuroendocrinology*
    37, 248-257.
11. Bjorklund, A. (1967). *Life Sci.* 6, 2103-2110.
12. Wingstraud, K.G. (1966). *In* "The Pituitary Gland"(Eds
    G.W. Harris and B.T. Donovan). pp. 1-27. Butter-
    worths, London.
13. Jackson, S. and Lowry, P.J. (1980). *J. Endocrinol.* 86,
    205-219.
14. Thody, A.J. (1980). "The MSH Peptides" Academic Press,
    London.
15. Swaab, D.F. and Martin, T.J. (1981). *In* "Peptides of
    the Pars Intermedia". Ciba Foundation Symposium '81.
    Pitman Medical, London pp. 196-217.
16. Challis, J.R.G. and Torosis, J.D. (1977) *Nature* 269,
    818-819.
17. Rudman, D., Hollins, B.M., Lewis, N.C. and Chawla, R.K.
    (1980). *J. Clin. Invest.* 65, 822-828.
18. Vinson, G.P., Whitehouse, B.J., Dell, A., Etienne, T.
    and Morris, H.R. (1980). *Nature* 284, 464-467.
19. Das, S., Edwardson, J.A., Hughes, D. and McDermott, J.R
    (1982). *In* "Neuroendocrinology of Vasopressin, Cort-
    icoliberin and Opiomelanocortins" (Eds A.J. Baert-
    schi and J.J. Dreifuss) Academic Press, pp. 33-41.
20. Beloff-Chain, A., Morton, J., Dunmore, S., Taylor, G.W.
    and Morris, H.R. (1983). *Nature* 301, 255-258.

21. Vale, W., Speiss, J., Rivier, C. and Rivier, J. (1981). *Science* 213, 1394-1396.
22. Vale, W., Vaughan, J., Smith, M., Yamamoto, G., Rivier, J. and Rivier, C. (1983). *Endocrinology* 113, 1121-1131.
23. Garren, L.D., Gill, G.N., Masui, H. and Walton, G.M. (1971). *Recent Prog. Horm. Res.* 27, 433-474.
24. Hechter, O. and Braun, T.H. (1971). *In* "Structure-Activity Relationships of Protein and Polypeptide Hormones". Part 1. (Eds M. Margoules and Greenwood, F) Exerpta Medica, pp. 212-227.
25. Matsuoka, H., Mulrow, P.J. and Li, C.H. (1980). *Nature* 209, 307-308.
26. Pedersen, R.C. and Brownie, A.C. (1980). *Proc. Natl. Acad. Sci.* 77, 2239-2243.
27. Al-Dujaili, E.A.S., Hope, J., Estivariz, F.E., Lowry, P.J. and Edwards, C.R.W. (1981). *Nature* 291, 156-159.
28. Al-Dujaili, E.A.S., Williams, B.C., Edwards, C.R.W., Salacinski, P.R. and Lowry, P.J. (1982). *Biochem.J.* 204, 301-305.
29. Perersen, R.C., Brownie, A.C. and Ling, N. (1980). *Science* 208, 1044-1045.
30. Scott, A.P. and Lowry, P.J. (1974). *Biochem. J.* 139, 593-602.
31. Bloomfield, G.A., Scott, A.P., Lowry, P.J., Gilkes, J.J.H. and Rees, L.H. (1974). *Nature* 252, 492-493.
32. Estivariz, F.E., Hope, J., McLean, C. and Lowry, P.J. (1980). *Biochem. J.* 191, 125-132.
33. Estivariz, F.E., Iturriza, F., McLean, C., Hope, J. and Lowry, P.J. (1982). *Nature* 297, 419-422.
34. Lowry, P.J., Silas, L., Linton, E.A., McLean, C. and Estivariz, F.E. (1983). *Nature* 306, 70-72.
35. Dallman, M.F., Engleland, W.C. and Mebride, M.H. (1977). *Ann. N.Y. Acad. Sci.* 297, 373-390.

CLINICAL STUDIES WITH GROWTH HORMONE RELEASING FACTOR

M.O. Thorner*, W.S. Evans*, M.L. Vance*,
R.M. Blizzard*, A.D. Rogol*, D.L. Kaiser*,
R. Furlanetto**, L.A. Frohman[+], J. Rivier[++] and W. Vale[++]

*University of Virginia, Charlottesville, VA 22908 USA,

**The Children's Hospital of Philadelphia, PA 19104, USA,

[+]University of Cincinnati, Cincinnati, OH 45267 USA,

[++]Peptide Biology Laboratory, The Salk Institute,
San Diego, CA 92138-9216, USA

INTRODUCTION

We have previously described in detail the presentation
and results of the study of a patient who harbored a
pancreatic tumor secreting a growth hormone (GH) releasing
factor (GRF) (1). This 40 amino acid-containing peptide
(hpGRF-40) was extracted, isolated, sequenced and a
synthetic replicate produced (2,3). A 44 amino acid peptide
(hpGRF-44) was identified from another pancreatic tumor and
subsequently synthesized (4). Convincing immunological,
biochemical and genetic information has now confirmed that
human hypothalamic GH releasing hormone (GHRH) is identical
to human pancreatic tumor GRF(s) and has approximately 70%
homology with rat hypothalamic GHRH (5-8). We now review
our first 13 months of clinical experience with GRF.
   The studies were performed with the approval of the Food
and Drug Administration and the Human Investigation
Committees of our respective institutions. We have used
hpGRF-40 which was synthesized and formulated as previously
described (2,9). Our initial studies were performed in
normal subjects, in adults with GH deficiency, and in
children with short stature.
   The availability of synthetic GRF for clinical use has
allowed us and others to investigate some aspects of the
physiology of GH secretion. We believe that these *in vivo*
studies together with *in vitro* studies may yield new and

DOPAMINE AND NEUROENDOCRINE   Copyright©1985 by Academic Press Inc. (London) Ltd.
ACTIVE SUBSTANCES   All rights of reproduction in any form reserved
ISBN 0 12 209045 4

effective therapies including those for GH deficient children and possibly for the prevention of the long term complications of diabetes mellitus thought to be due to GH excess. In addition, new approaches to the diagnosis and treatment of acromegaly may be forthcoming.

STUDIES IN NORMAL MEN

Our first study in humans, which consisted of administration of 1 ug/kg body weight hpGRF-40 given as an intravenous (i.v.) bolus (9), was followed by a study of the dose response relationship (10). hpGRF-40 selectively stimulated GH secretion with serum GH concentrations increasing within 5 minutes, and reaching a peak between 30 and 60 minutes (20.4 $\pm$ 6.5 ng/ml compared with 2.1 $\pm$ 0.1 ng/ml after placebo; mean $\pm$ SEM). Serum levels of prolactin, thyrotropin (TSH), luteinizing hormone (LH) and corticotropin (measured indirectly through plasma cortisol) were not increased after administration of hpGRF-40. Similarly, the concentrations of blood glucose, plasma insulin, glucagon, pancreatic polypeptide, cholecystokinin, gastrin, gastric inhibitory peptide, motilin, and somatostatin were unaffected by hpGRF-40. There were no changes in blood pressure, pulse rate, or body temperature, and no side-effects were noted.

A dose response relationship was next determined by documenting the effect of graded doses of hpGRF-40 on GH release in healthy men (10). Mean peak increments in GH following vehicle and various doses of hpGRF-40 were 1.13, 11.4, 14.6, 17.01, 14.45, and 15.6 ng/ml after vehicle and 0.1, 0.33, 1, 3.3, and 10 ug/kg hpGRF-40 given as an i.v. bolus, respectively (Figure 1). Peak values were observed 30 to 60 minutes after administration of hpGRF-40. There was considerable variability in response among individual subjects and no dose-response relationship between the doses and maximal GH levels achieved was observed. However, the higher doses of 3.3 and 10 ug/kg were associated with a more prolonged, biphasic pattern of GH release. Side effects of facial flushing of less than 5 minutes duration occurred in 4 of 6 subjects who received 3.3 ug/kg and in all 6 who received 10 ug/kg of hpGRF-40. No changes in serum glucose, LH, TSH, prolactin, plasma cortisol or 8 enteropancreatic hormones were observed following hpGRF-40. There were small increases in serum somatomedin C levels 24 hours after administration of various doses of hpGRF-40 in 11 of 13 studies. Mean plasma immunoreactive GRF levels measured 5 minutes after injection were 0.09, 2.0, 4.86, 23.90, and 66.6 ng/ml after 0.1, 0.33, 1, 3.3 and 10 ug/kg of hpGRF-40,

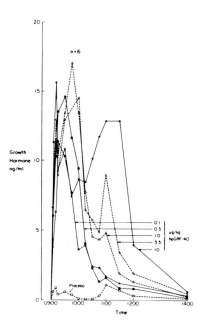

Fig. 1. Mean changes in serum GH (ng/ml) over baseline after vehicle, 0.1, 0.33, 1.0, 3.3 and 10 ug/kg hpGRF-40 i.v. bolus in normal men. The doses of 3.3 and 10 ug/kg result in a second GH peak approximately two hours after administration (biphasic response). N = 11 for vehicle; N = 6 for 0.1, 0.33, 1.0 and 3.3 ug/kg, and N = 5 for 10 ug/kg dose of hpGRF-40. Reproduced from Vance et al. (10) with permission.

respectively. Serum GH responses after insulin-induced hypoglycemia were compared to GH responses following hpGRF-40. Comparable GH stimulation occurred with both provocative tests. Mean ($+$ SEM) peak GH after insulin was 20.2 ± 1.04 ng/ml and 20.9 ± 3.16 following hpGRF-40. Our studies are similar to those reported subsequently using hpGRF-44 by Wood et al. (11), Rosenthal et al. (12), and Gelato et al. (13). However, in those studies no consistent dose response relationship was observed.

STUDIES IN NORMAL WOMEN

Having shown in normal men that hpGRF-40 could stimulate GH secretion, we next examined its effects in normal women (Evans et al. submitted for publication). We administered hpGRF-40 (3.33 ug/kg; test day) or an equivalent volume of vehicle (control day) as an i.v. bolus at 0900 h to 5 normal subjects. All women were studied during the early follicular, late follicular, and mid-luteal phases of the menstrual cycle. Serum concentrations of GH, prolactin, LH and follicle-stimulating hormone (FSH) were measured at intervals between 0800–1200 h. Serum somatomedin C concentrations were obtained prior to and 24 hours following administration of vehicle or hpGRF-40. Within 1–3 minutes following injection of hpGRF-40 all women described warmth which was localized to the head and neck and exhibited facial flushing. No changes in pulse rate or blood pressure were noted. Median maximal levels of serum GH (ng/ml; control vs test day) were higher following hpGRF-40 during the early follicular (6.2 vs 23.1; p=0.0216), late follicular (5.4 vs 22.7; p=0.0216) and luteal (3.2 vs 16.8; p=0.0122) phases of the menstrual cycle. When expressed as change from baseline, median integrated serum GH levels (ng/ml/h) were higher following hpGRF-40 than control values during the early follicular (1.18 vs 13.5; control vs test day) and luteal (-2.22 vs 5.16) phases of the menstrual cycle (p=0.0122). Although higher in 4 of 5 subjects, median integrated serum GH levels were not increased following hpGRF-40 during the late follicular phase (1.44 vs 4.53; p=0.17). Serum somatomedin C values 24 hours after hpGRF-40 were higher compared to those 24 hours after vehicle at all stages of the menstrual cycle. hpGRF-40 did not stimulate the release of prolactin, LH, or FSH. These studies suggest that hpGRF-40 selectively stimulates the release of biologically active GH in women but that, at the dose tested, hpGRF-40-stimulated GH release does not vary as a function of the gonadal hormone environment.

ROUTES OF ADMINISTRATION

Since GRF for therapeutic use will probably require administration several times each day, parenteral administration may interfere with its utility. We thus undertook a preliminary investigation on the effects of intranasal administration of hpGRF-40 (14). hpGRF-40 (30 ug/kg; test day) or an equivalent volume of vehicle alone (control day) was administered to 6 normal men at 0900 h. Immunoreactive GH was measured in serum obtained at intervals between 0800-1200 h. Mean (± SEM) integrated serum levels of GH (ng/ml/h) prior to and following administration of vehicle were not different (1.27 ± 0.57 vs 0.87 ± 0.28; p = 0.54). However, following hpGRF-40 administration, GH levels increased significantly (0.53 ± 0.03 vs 2.88 ± 0.75; p=0.022). Peak levels of serum GH were detected within 30 minutes following hpGRF-40. Except for mild burning of the nasal mucosa reported by one subject, no side effects were noted. We have subsequently investigated the dose response relationship of intranasal hpGRF-40 administration (3-100 ug/kg) and GH secretion. Only the 30 ug/kg and 100 ug/kg doses of hpGRF-40 stimulated GH secretion when administered by this route. The dose required to stimulate GH secretion by the intranasal route was extremely large thus precluding use of the peptide by this route using this formulation.

We have therefore administered hpGRF-40 (1-10 ug/kg) subcutaneously. Our results demonstrate a dose response relationship between hpGRF-40 and GH release over this dose range. Although 1 ug/kg hpGRF-40 administered subcutaneously appears to stimulate GH release, the 3.3 and 10 ug/kg doses were associated with greater and more prolonged increases.

PHARMACOKINETICS OF hpGRF-40

Most hypothalamic hormones are small peptides with very short half-lives. It was therefore important to define the pharmacokinetics of GRF in the human. Using two different techniques we investigated the metabolic clearance rate and plasma disappearance rate in normal men by single injection and constant infusion techniques (15). Immunoreactive GRF levels were measured by radioimmunoassay using an extracted plasma specimen with hpGRF-40 as radioiodionated tracer, an antibody raised against hpGRF(1-20), and a second antibody separation method.

We determined in normal adult male subjects the metabolic clearance rate (MCR) and plasma disappearance rate ($T_{1/2}$) of hpGRF-40. Single i.v. injections of 1, 3.3, and 10 ug/kg hpGRF-40 were administered. Plasma immunoreactive (IR) GRF levels were measured during the subsequent 180 minutes, and biexponential curve analysis was performed. Graded dose constant infusions of hpGRF-40 at rates of 1, 3.3, 10, and 33 ng/kg/min were administered and the MCR calculated from measurement of steady state plasma IR-GRF levels at each infusion rate. The post-infusion disappearance rate was determined by linear regression analysis of plasma IR-GRF levels during the 120-minute period after cessation of the infusion.

The calculated MCR ($1/m^2/d$) during the single injection study was 194 ± 17.5 and was not significantly different from the calculated value during the constant infusion study (202 ± 16). The disappearance rate during the single injection study was subdivided into two linear phases: an initial equilibration phase (7.6 ± 1.2 min) and a subsequent elimination phase (51.8 ± 5.4 min). The latter was similar to the linear disappearance rate observed (41.3 ± 3.0 min) after cessation of the constant infusion. The chromatographic and biologic characteristics of plasma IR-GRF, 30 minutes after injection, were similar to those of synthetic hpGRF-40.

STUDIES IN GH DEFICIENT ADULTS

In our initial study hpGRF-40, 10 ug/kg, was administered intravenously to 6 normal young men and 12 adult patients who had presented in childhood with GH deficiency (7 patients had isolated GH deficiency, 4 had multiple anterior pituitary hormone deficiencies, and 1 had Hand-Schuller-Christian [HSC] disease) (16). hpGRF-40 administration increased serum GH concentrations in all normal subjects and in 3 of 7 patients with isolated GH deficiency and in the 1 with HSC disease; however, the mean serum GH concentration in the patients who responded was less than that of the normal subjects. Serum somatomedin C concentrations were increased 24 hours after a single dose of hpGRF-40 in 8 of 10 patients with GH deficiency. In agreement with these findings were the studies of Wood et al. (11), Grossman et al. (17), and Takano et al. (18).

More recently we have studied 6 adult subjects who presented in childhood with idiopathic GH deficiency by challenging them with 10 ug/kg hpGRF-40 i.v. bolus prior to and following 5 days of treatment with 0.33 ug/kg hpGRF-40 administered i.v. every 3 hours (19). Serum GH levels were monitored daily for 90 minutes after the 0800 h doses of 0.33 ug/kg hpGRF-40 and serum somatomedin C was measured at 0800 and 2000 h. In addition plasma levels of cholesterol, high density lipoprotein (HDL)-cholesterol, and triglycerides were measured daily at 0800 h. Three hours after the last 0.33 ug/kg dose, all subjects were rechallenged with 10 ug/kg hpGRF-40. In response to the initial 10 ug/kg challenge with hpGRF-40, and although serum GH levels rose in 4 of the 7 subjects, the mean maximum GH level was no different from that after vehicle alone. Within 12 hours after initiation of the intermittent administration of hpGRF-40, mean ($\pm$ SEM) somatomedin C had risen by 0.1 ± 0.05 U/ml and at the end of the 5 day period had increased from 0.24 ± 0.07 to 0.78 ± 0.32 U/ml (Figure 2). In response to the second challenge with 10 ug/kg hpGRF-40 serum GH levels rose in 3 of the 4 subjects who initially failed to respond or had a $<$ 1 ng/ml response (Figure 3). The increase in serum GH was greater in 1 of the 2 subjects who had responded to the first dose. In addition, unlike the first dose, the mean maximal serum GH level achieved in response to second 10 ug/kg dose of hpGRF-40 was higher when compared to vehicle ($p=0.031$). Although there was no statistically significant change during the 5 day period in plasma cholesterol, HDL-cholesterol, or triglycerides, the latter exhibited a strong trend towards increased levels. Thus

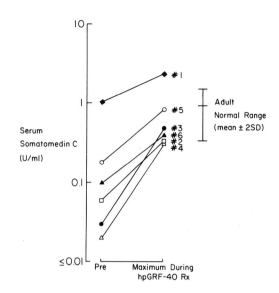

Fig. 2. Serum
somatomedin C
levels (U/ml) be-
fore and maximum
levels observed
during 5 days of
intermittent pul-
satile hpGRF-40
administration.
Note logarithmic
scale. Reproduced
from Borges et al.
(18) with per-
mission.

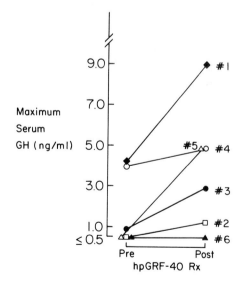

Fig. 3. Maximum
serum levels (ng/
ml) in 6 adults
with idiopathic GH
deficiency after
i.v. bolus hpGRF-
40 (10 ug/kg) be-
fore and the ter-
mination of 5 days
of hpGRF 40 0.33
ug/kg i.v. bolus
given every 3 h.
Reproduced from
Borges et al. (18)
with permission.

these data show that 5 days of intermittent hpGRF-40
administration augments GH secretion in some adults with GH
deficiency, suggesting that the somatotropes that are
present in idiopathic GH deficiency may be primed by
hpGRF-40. The rise in serum somatomedin C to normal levels
after multiple injections of hpGRF-40 is encouraging, since
circulating levels of somatomedin C may be more important
than the increase in immunoreactive GH levels as an index of
response for induction of linear growth. The demonstration
of biological effects of hpGRF-40 in all 6 subjects, without
any serious adverse effects, suggests that hpGRF-40 has
promise in the treatment of GH deficiency.

STUDIES IN CHILDREN WITH SHORT STATURE

    Forty children with short stature were evaluated for GH
reserve following pharmacological tests and after a single
i.v. bolus injection of hpGRF-40. These children were
grouped into four diagnostic categories: (1) idiopathic GH
deficiency (IGHD); (2) organic hypopituitarism; (3) intra-
uterine growth retardation (IUGR); and (4) constitutional
delay of growth (CD), by standard clinical criteria and
physiological and pharmacological tests of GH reserve. A
fifth category, unclassified by these criteria, was also
included.
    Subjects were tested on two consecutive days: (1) follow-
ing the intravenous administration of L-arginine (0.5 mg/kg
over 30 min) and the oral administration of L-dihydroxy-
phenylalanine (L-DOPA, 9 mg/kg), and (2) following the
administration of hpGRF-40, 3.3 ug/kg, as an intravenous
bolus.
    The GH deficient patients in categories 1 and 2 failed to
raise their circulating GH concentrations to more than 7
ng/ml following the arginine-L-DOPA test, but some showed
marked GH responses following hpGRF-40 administration. As a
group, however, the lowest responses (mean $\pm$ SE) to the
releasing factor were noted in the organic hypopituitary
(3.4 $\pm$ 1.1 ng/ml) and in the IGHD (8.2 $\pm$ 2.4 ng/ml)
categories. All children in the IUGR, CD, and unclassified
groups responded briskly to hpGRF-40, although there was
wide variation of the peak GH level (5 to more than 25
ng/ml).
    These data indicate that hpGRF-40 can be employed to
evaluate GH reserve in short children and may be useful in
the diagnosis of hypothalamic-pituitary disorders. The
ultimate test of the utility of hpGRF-40 in children with GH
deficiency or short stature is the therapeutic response

(growth) when compared to the presently available natural or synthetic GH preparations.

With this in mind we have recently started to treat 2 children with idiopathic GH deficiency with hpGRF-40 administered subcutaneously every 3 hours. These children have been treated for approximately 8 weeks now. They have tolerated the treatment well and it has been associated with a rise in serum somatomedin C, and priming of the somatotroph. However, it is too early to tell whether it has led to acceleration in linear growth.

CONCLUSIONS

In the 13 months since synthetic hpGRF has been available for clinical use it has been determined that it is a specific secretagogue (except in unusual circumstances) for GH secretion; i.e., it fails to affect the secretion of the other anterior pituitary hormones or of at least 8 entero-pancreatic hormones. The peptide is effective in stimulating GH secretion when administered intravenously, subcutaneously, or intranasally although at least 20 and 100 fold the effective intravenous dose is required for the subcutaneous and intranasal routes, respectively. Doses as low as 0.1 ug/kg i.v. produce maximal GH secretion although higher doses have a more prolonged duration of action.

The pharmacokinetics of GRF are unlike those of thyrotropin releasing hormone (TRH), gonadotropin releasing hormone (GnRH), or somatostatin, but similar to those of corticotropin releasing factor (CRF) which is of similar molecular size having 41 amino acids.

The ability of hpGRF to stimulate GH secretion in only a minority of GH deficient adults, but somatomedin C in a majority, and the high proportion of children of short stature who respond to hpGRF, make it likely that hpGRF may have a role in therapy of GH deficiency. This is also suggested by the longer term administration of GRF in the GH hormone deficient adults and the very preliminary data in the GH deficient children. The role of hpGRF in other human disease is more speculative but may include the treatment of negative nitrogen balance seen in the aging process; it may also have a role in the treatment of short stature in the absence of GH deficiency.

In the coming months we hope to be able to determine whether hpGRF therapy is effective in stimulating linear growth in GH deficient children.

ACKNOWLEDGEMENTS

    We thank Dr. Michael J. Cronin for helpful assistance;
Mrs Sandra W. Jackson, Ms Fotini Beziriannidis, Mrs Jean
Chitwood, Pattie Hellmann, Ms Kathryn Wolf and the staff of
the Clinical Research Center for their help; the staff of
the laboratories at our respective institutions for technical
assistance; Mrs Donna Harris and Mrs Ina Hofland for assistance in the preparation of the manuscript, and the Pituitary
Hormone Distribution Program of the National Institute of
Arthritis, Diabetes, Digestive and Kidney Diseases for RIA
reagents for measurements of human GH and LH. These studies
were supported in part by US Public Health Service research
grants: General Clinical Research Grant RR-847; HD-13197 and
AM-32632 (M.O.T.); CIA 1-K03-HD-00439 (W.S.E.); 1R23-HD-17120
(M.L.V.); AM-26741, AM-209117, AA-03504, and HD-13527 (P.B.L.)
and AM-30667 (L.A.F.).

REFERENCES

1. Thorner, M.O., Perryman, R.L., Cronin, M.J., Rogol, A.D.,
        Draznin, M., Johanson, A., Vale, W., Horvath, E. and
        Kovacs, K. (1982). *J. Clin. Invest.* 70, 965-977.
2. Rivier, J., Spiess, J., Thorner, M.O. and Vale, W.
        (1982). *Nature* 300, 276-278.
3. Spiess, J., Rivier, J., Thorner, M.O. and Vale, W. (1982).
        Biochemistry 21, 6037-6040.
4. Guillemin, R., Brazeau, P., Bohlen, P., Esch, F., Ling,
        N. and Wehrenberg, W. (1982). *Science* 218, 585-587.
5. Rivier, J., Spiess, J. and Vale, W. (1984). *In* "Pro-
        ceedings of Eighth American Peptide Symposium" (Eds
        V.J. Hruby and D.H. Rich), in press, Pierce Chemical
        Company.
6. Gubler, U., Monahan, J.J., Lomedico, P.T., Bhatt, R.S.,
        Collier, K.J., Hoffman, B.J., Bohlen, P., Esch, F.,
        Ling, N., Zeytin, F., Brazeau, P., Poonian, M.S. and
        Gage, L.P. (1983). *Proc. Natl. Acad. Sci.* 80, 4311-4314
7. Mayo, K.E., Vale, W., Rivier, J., Rosenfeld, G. and Evans,
        R.M. (1983). *Nature* 306, 86-88.
8. Spiess, J., Rivier, J. and Vale, W. (1983). *Nature* 303,
        532-535.
9. Thorner, M.O., Rivier, J., Spiess, J., Borges, J.L.C.,
        Vance, M.L., Bloom, S.R., Rogol, A.D., Cronin, M.J.,
        Kaiser, D.L., Evans, W.S., Webster, J.D., MacLeod, R.M.
        and Vale, W. (1983). *Lancet* i, 24-28.
10. Vance, M.L., Borges, J.L.C., Kaiser, D.L., Evans, W.S.,
        Furlanetto, R., Thominet, J.L., Frohman, L.A., Rogol,

    A.D., MacLeod, R.M., Bloom, S., Rivier, J., Vale, W.
    and Thorner, M.O. (1984). *J. Clin. Endocrinol. Metab.*
    58, 838-844.
11. Wood, S.M., Ch'ng, J.L.C., Adams, E.F., Webster, J.D.,
    Joplin, G.F., Maschiter, K. and Bloom, S.R. (1983).
    Br. Med. J. 286, 1687-1691.
12. Rosenthal, S.M., Schriock, E.A., Kaplan, S.L., Guillemin,
    R. and Grumbach, M.M. (1983). *J. Clin. Endocrinol.
    Metab.* 57, 677-679.
13. Gelato, M.C., Pescovits, O., Cassorla, F., Loriaux, D.L.
    and Merriam, G.R. (1983). *J. Clin. Endocrinol. Metab.*
    57, 674-676.
14. Evans, W.S., Borges, J.L.C., Kaiser, D.L., Vance, M.L.,
    Sellers, R.P., MacLeod, R.M., Vale, W., Rivier, J.
    and Thorner, M.O. (1983). *J. Clin. Endocrinol. Metab.*
    57, 1081-1083.
15. Frohman, L.A., Thominet, J.L., Webb, C.B., Vance, M.L.,
    Uderman, H., Rivier, J., Vale, W. and Thorner, M.O.
    (1984). *J. Clin. Invest.* 73, 1304-1311.
16. Borges, J.L.C., Blizzard, R.M., Gelato, M.C., Furlanetto,
    R., Rogol, A.D., Evans, W.S., Vance, M.L., Kaiser, D.L.,
    MacLeod, R.M., Merriam, G.R., Loriaux, D.L., Spiess, J.,
    Rivier, J., Vale, W. and Thorner, M.O. (1983). *Lancet*
    ii, 119-124.
17. Grossman, A., Savage, M.O., Wass, J.A.H., Lytras, N.,
    Sueiras- Diaz, J., Coy, D.H. and Besser, G.M. (1983).
    Lancet ii, 137-138.
18. Takano, K., Hizuka, N., Shizume, K., Asakawa, K., Miyakawa,
    M., Hirose, N., Shibasaki, T. and Ling, N.C. (1984).
    J. Clin. Endocrinol. Metab. 58, 236-241.
19. Borges, J.L.C., Blizzard, R.M., Evans, W.S., Furlanetto,
    R., Rogol, A.D., Kaiser, D.L., Rivier, J., Vale, W.
    and Thorner, M.O. (1984). *J. Clin. Endocrinol. Metab.*
    59, 1-6.

CLINICAL EVALUATION OF CRF

O.A. Müller, J. Schopohl, G.K. Stalla and K. von Werder

Medizinische Klinik Innenstadt
University of Munich, 8000 Munich 2, FRG

INTRODUCTION

Since the characterization of a 41-residue Ovine Corticotropin Releasing Factor (oCRF) by Vale *et al.* in 1981 (1),
the scarcity of human data obtained with this peptide contrasts with the great number of experimental animal studies.
The biological activity of synthetic oCRF in humans was first
demonstrated by Grossman *et al.* (2) and Müller *et al.* (3).
Later on, the usefulness of this substance in the evaluation
of diseases involving the hypothalamo-pituitary-adrenal axis
was amply demonstrated (3,4,5,6).
    The aim of the present work was the study of a CRF-stimu-
lation test in normal volunteers as compared with patients
with diseases affecting central control of the adrenal glands.
In addition, a specific radioimmunoassay for oCRF was developed, allowing the measurement of circulating concentrations
of the peptide subsequent to its intravenous administration.
This procedure was established in order to investigate the
plasma kinetics of oCRF in an attempt to clarify the heterogeneity of ACTH responses to this substance reported in the
literature (7).

MATERIALS AND METHODS

CRF-Standards and Administration

Synthetic ovine and human CRF were obtained from Bachem
Inc. (Bubendorf, Switzerland), or from Henning GmbH (Berlin,
FRG). CRF was lyophilized in sterile ampoules in different
dosages. Before intravenous administration the substance was
dissolved in 1 ml 0.02% HCl in 0.9% saline.

Test Protocol and Subjects

Informed consent was obtained from volunteers and patients
before entering the trial. CRF-administration (oCRF or hCRF)
was performed between 8.30 and 9.30 a.m. after an overnight
fast. A cubital vein was cannulated and kept patent with an
intravenous saline infusion. Blood samples were obtained 15,30,
45, 60 , 90 and 120 minutes after intravenous administration
of 50, 100 or 200 ug CRF.

Hormone Measurements

ACTH was measured by radioimmunoassay using N-terminal
specific antibodies after silic acid plasma extraction as
described earlier (8,9). Synthetic human 1-39 ACTH (Ciba-
Geigy) served as the standard (pg/ml). Blood specimens for
ACTH were collected on ice in tubes containing EDTA and Tras-
ylol and were immediately centrifuged and kept frozen at
-80°C until analyzed (normal values: 15-50 pg/ml). CRF was
measured by a specific radioimmunoassay using synthetic oCRF
as the standard and for immunization (details in 11,12).
Cortisol was measured by radioimmunoassay without prior extraction as described previously (10) (normal values: 5-20
ug/dl). The intraassay coefficient of variation for ACTH was
less than 10% and for cortisol less than 5%. The interassay
variation for ACTH was less than 18% and for cortisol less
than 11%.

RESULTS

No relevant side effects were observed after injection of
oCRF or hCRF (3,4,12). In healthy volunteers the increases
in ACTH and cortisol were dose-dependent after 50 and 100 ug
but no further increments were observed after 200 ug. There
was a clearcut relationship between the maximal CRF-levels
measured 15 minutes after oCRF injection and the injected
dosage of oCRF. The administration of the homologous human
CRF did not lead to a different ACTH- and cortisol-response
in normal subjects compared with the heterologous oCRF. In
contrast to the results with oCRF, ACTH- and cortisol-responses
to 50 ug hCRF were indistinguishable from the responses to
100 ug hCRF, underlining the remarkable heterogeneity of
CRF stimulated ACTH-secretion (7,11,12).
Fig. 1 shows first results in 3 normal volunteers after a
bolus injections of 100 ug hCRF given at 9 and 12 o'clock in
the morning, at 3 o'clock in the afternoon, and again at

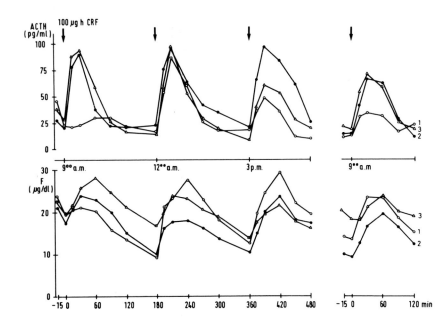

Fig. 1. Repeated bolus injections of 100 ug hCRF in three healthy volunteers: effect on plasma ACTH and cortisol (F).

9 o'clock the next day. In all 3 volunteers, comparable ACTH-
and cortisol-increases after each stimulation were recorded.
Fig. 2 shows the responses to the same stimulation followed
by an infusion of hCRF at a rate of 100 ug/h for three hours.
At the end of the follow-up period another *bolus* injection
of 100 ug was administered. The first administration of hCRF
led to typical ACTH- and cortisol-increases. ACTH- and cortisol plasma levels remained elevated throughout the CRF infusion. The next CRF bolus injection did not lead to a further
increase in two volunteers and only to small increment in one
subject.

In Patients with disturbances of the hypothalamo-pituitary
adrenal axis, CRF stimulation tests with 100 ug oCRF were performed. It has been previously shown that oCRF is not a diagnostic tool but can be useful in the differential diagnosis
of proven Cushing's syndrome (4). In patients with ACTH-dependent Cushing's disease normal or elevated basal ACTH-levels
were significantly higher after stimulation with CRF compared
with normal controls. The pattern of cortisol secretion following CRF-administration corresponded to that of ACTH secretion
in these patients. In one subject with ectopic ACTH-syndrome

extremely elevated ACTH and cortisol plasma levels did not
change significantly after CRF-administration (4). In contrast, patients with unilateral adrenal adenoma or carcinoma
had suppressed ACTH-levels which did not rise after CRF-administration (4,12).

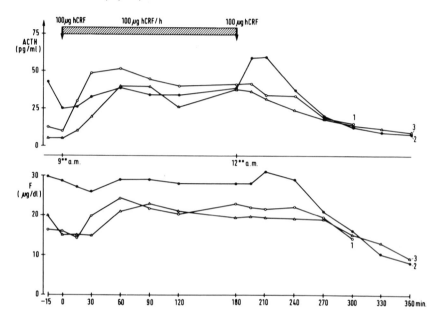

*Fig. 2. Bolus injection of 100 ug hCRF followed by infusion
of 100 ug hCRF/hour for three hours, again followed by another
bolus injection of 100 ug hCRF.*

No significant change in cortisol-secretion could be observed.
Fig. 3 shows the significantly greater increase in ACTH-secretion induced by 100 ug oCRF in 14 patients with ACTH-dependent Cushing's disease compared with healthy volunteers.
In contrast, the suppressed ACTH release recorded in 6 patients with autonomous cortisol hypersecretion caused by an
adrenal adenoma or carcinoma did not react to oCRF.

A blunted ACTH and cortisol increase to CRF stimulation
after selective adenomectomy in patients with ACTH-dependent
Cushing's disease was first shown by Orth *et al.* (6). Similar
response patterns were observed among our patients (3,12) but
a number of them also reacted to a oCRF challenge with normal
ACTH and cortisol elevations (12).

The results of stimulation with oCRF are different following unilateral adrenalectomy due to a cortisol-producing
adenoma or carcinoma. Thus, the absence of ACTH and cortisol

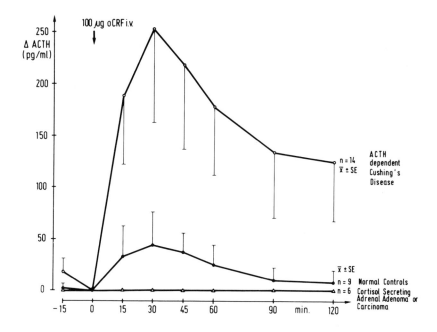

Fig. 3. ACTH-response after CRF-stimulation with 100 μg oCRF in 14 patients with ACTH-dependent Cushing's disease and in 6 patients with autonomous cortisol-secretion due to an adrenal adenoma or carcinoma.

responses to CRF are commonly encounteres subsequent to tumor removal (3,12). ACTH sensitivity is the first to appear in the postoperative stage (12). Fig. 4 shows the response patterns to oCRF recorded in the same two subjects at different intervals after unilateral adrenalectomy because of an adenoma or carcinoma. One patient (left panel) fails to react to oCRF shortly after surgery. One and a half years later, an adequate ACTH response is recorded but cortisol remains subnormal due to atrophy of the contralateral adrenal. In the other subject an andrenal carcinoma was found. Early post-surgery ACTH secretion remains suppressed by the abnormally elevated plasma cortisol maintained by a lung metastasis. A twelve month treatment period with o,p'-DDD substantially reduced plasma cortisol and recovery of the corticotrop response to oCRF is clearly demonstrable, thus documenting the positive response to adrenolytic therapy.

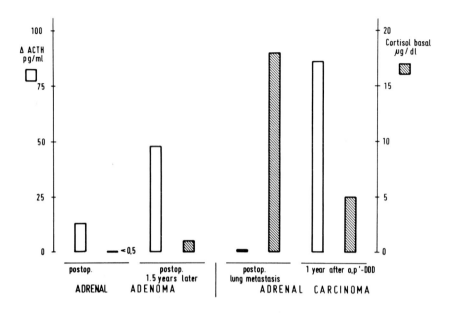

*Fig. 4. oCRF-stimulation-test at different times in two pa-
tients with operated autonomous cortisol-producing adrenal
adenoma or carcinoma.*

   The response to CRF in Cushing's syndrome induced by long-
term administration of exogenous glucocorticoids is quite
variable. In patients receiving high daily doses of dexamethasone there was no or little reaction observed, whereas subjects
receiving 10 mg prednisolone on alternate days exhibited an
ACTH response pattern similar to that recorded in normal individuals. Only these patients showed concomittant increments
in plasma cortisol (12). In three patients with ACTH-dependent
Cushing's disease who were treated daily with 8 mg dexamethasone, a marked suppression of ACTH and cortisol secretion was
recorded. In addition, the administration of dexamethasone
can negatively influence the ACTH response to CRF (Fig. 5).
This finding points to the pituitary as the main site of
corticosteroid action. The CRF-stimulation test can be advan-
tageous in the differential diagnosis of secondary adrenal
insufficiency. Thus, an adequate ACTH response would localize
the primary deffect in the hypothalamus whereas lack of response would reflect primary pituitary alteration (12).

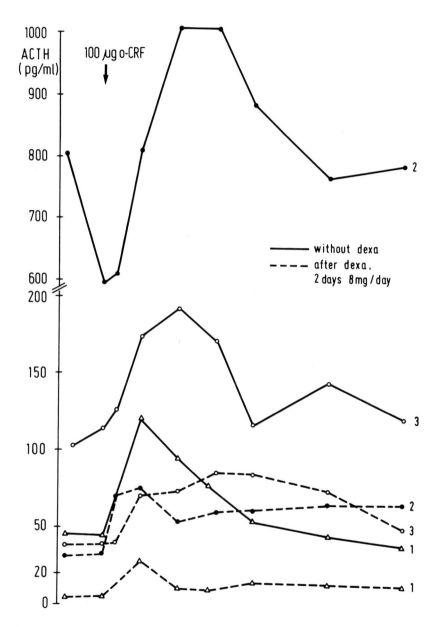

Fig. 5. ACTH-levels after 100 g oCRF in 3 patients with ACTH-dependent Cushing's disease without dexamethasone and after dexamethasone (8 mg/day over 2 days).

RESPONSE OF GH AND ACTH TO HYPOGLYCEMIA, GRF, AND CRF IN PATIENTS WITH SUPRASELLAR TUMOURS

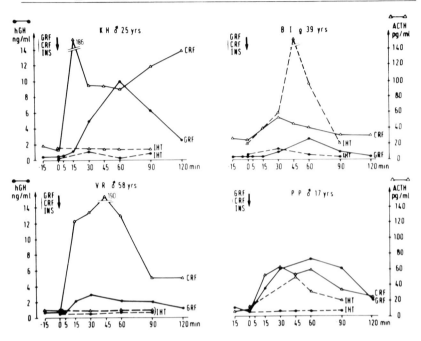

*Fig. 6. ACTH- and hGH-levels after insulin-induced hypoglyce-
mia, CRF- and GRF-stimulation in 4 patients with suprasellar
tumors.*

Fig. 6 depicts the result of a combined stimulation test,
insulin-CRF-GRF, in 4 patients with suprasellar tumors. No
ACTH and GH elevations to insulin were recorded in a dysgermi-
noma patient (K.H.), but responses to CRF and GRF were preserved. A similar reaction was observed in another patient
with suprasellar metastasis (V.R.). In two patients with
craniopharyngiomas the GH plasma profile following insulin
was blunted, whereas somatotrops responded to GRF with substantial GH increments. ACTH release was unaffected further
documenting the increased resistance of corticotrops to ex-
pansive processes involving the hypothalamo-pituitary area.
These are typical response patterns now confirmed by the
authors in 10 cases of hypothalamic disease (14).

DISCUSSION

Previous experience has shown that the administration of synthetic oCRF leads to a rapid increase of ACTH and β-endorphin release which reaches peak plasma concentrations approximately 30 minutes after injection. Cortisol increases to a maximum within 60 minutes and remains above resting levels for at least 120 minutes (2,3,12). However, there is a marked heterogeneity in the ACTH and cortisol response patterns to CRF (2,3,7,12). Thus, Orth *et al.* (7) could only demonstrate a dose-effect relationship over a wide oCRF dosage range. Considering that a number of cardiovascular side effects have been recorded with oCRF doses above 100 ug (15), it is the authors' opinion that there is no advantage in using higher amounts of oCRF for clinical purposes. Indeed, the 100 ug dosage has proven to be effective as a diagnostic tool in conditions involving the hypothalamo-pituitary connections. In this context it should be mentioned that the newly introduced human CRF has failed to show any advantages in its clinical usefulness in comparison with the heterologous oCRF. Certainly, the lack of antigenicity of the human peptide will render it one of the most useful therapeutical tools of the future.

It has been proposed that the wide individual variation in the response pattern to a given CRF dose may be due to mechanical artefacts such as absorption to glass or tubing systems (7). However, measurement of specific oCRF radioimmunoactivity in plasma of subjects receiving graded doses of this peptide has revealed a close correlation between the administered amounts and plasma concentrations of oCRF excluding adsorption to the carrier systems as the cause. Other factors such as endogenous vasopressin release into the portal blood, which is known to influence ACTH secretion independently of CRF, may play a more relevant role (18,19). Also the type of stimulation used should be taken into consideration since insulin was found to induce a more marked ACTH release than CRF itself (unpublished results). This effect could also be mediated by arginine vasopressin or other centrally active substances.

The acute administration of oCRF represents a well tolerated and useful test in the differential diagnosis of hyper- or hypofunctional states of the hypothalamo-pituitary-adrenal axis. This procedure has proven to be very useful in the differential diagnosis of Cushing's syndrome (4,6). However, the ACTH response to CRF in Cushing's disease is quite variable, specially in cases with bilateral macro- and micronodular adrenocortical hyperplasia (20). The ACTH which is re-

leased following stimulation probably originates in the micro-
adenoma. The lack of responsiveness to oCRF subsequent to
selective tumor removal substantiates this theory (3,4,6,12).
Based on these experiences with CRF, we believe that this
peptide should replace lysine-vasopressin as a clinical test
in the diagnosis of Cushing's syndrome. In contrast to the
well known side effects that follow the intravenous administration of lysine-vasopressin, no serious reactions to the
injection of oCRF through the same route have been observed.
In patients on chronic corticosteroid therapy, the suppression
of the ACTH response to exogenous CRF depends on the dosage
and length of treatment. Therefore, this test may be indicative whether and when adrenal function is restored after
termination of corticosteroid treatment. This seem to influence central control of the adrenals at the level of the
pituitary since pre-treatment with dexamethasone will not
only reduce basal ACTH secretion but also the response to a
CRF challenge. These preliminary observations should be confirmed in future investigations.

The differential diagnosis between primary pituitary and
secondary hypothalamic failure is important for the management of patients with alterations of ACTH control. Results
of corticotrop stimulation with CRF in patients with secondary
adrenal insufficiency of unknown origin confirms the diagnostic value of the CRF test in the differentiation of this condition as previously proposed by the authors (3,12). Nevertheless, this procedure does not replace the insulin test
which documents the integrity of the complete hypothalamo-
pituitary-adrenal axis. The combination of both tests allows
one to differentiate between central and peripheral causes
of adrenal insufficiency even when there is an absence of recognizable anatomic abnormalities (12,17).

ACKNOWLEDGEMENTS

The skilled technical assistance of J. Hartwimmer is great-
fully acknowledged. - This study was supported by the
"Deutsche Forschungsgemeinschaft" (Mu 585/2-1).

REFERENCES

1. Vale, W., Spiess, J., Rivier, A. and Rivier, J. (1981).
    Science 213, 1394-1397.
2. Grossman, A., Nieuwenhuysen-Krusemann, A.G., Perry, L.,
    Tomlin, S., Schally, A.V., Coy, D.H., Rees, L.H.,
    Comaru-Schally, A.M. and Besser, G.M. (1982). *Lancet*
    I, 921-922.

3. Müller, O.A., Dörr, H.G., Hagen, B., Stalla, G.K. and
    von Werder, K. (1982). *Klin, Wschr.* 60, 1485-1491.
4. Müller, O.A., Stalla, G.K. and von Werder, K. (1983).
    J. Clin. Endocrinol. Metab. 57, 227-229.
5. Nakahara, M., Shibasaki, T., Shizume, K., Kiyosawa, Y.,
    Odagiri, E., Suda, T., Yamaguchi, H., Tsushima, T.,
    Demura, H., Maeda, T., Wakabayashi, I. and Ling, N.
    (1983). *J. Clin. Endocrinol. Metab.* 57, 963-968.
6. Orth, D.N., DeBold, C.R., DeCherney, G.S., Jackson, R.V.,
    Alexander, A.N., Rivier, J., Rivier, C., Spiess, J.
    and Vale, W. (1982). *J. Clin. Endocrinol. Metab.* 55,
    1017-1019.
7. Orth, D.N., Jackson, R.V., DeCherney, G.S., DeBold, C.R.,
    Alexander, A.N., Island, D.P. and Rivier, J. (1983).
    J. Clin. Invest. 71, 587-595.
8. Müller, O.A. (1980). *In* "ACTH im Plasma. Bestimmungs-
    methoden und klinische Bedeutung". Thieme-Cypothek,
    Stuttgart.
9. Müller, O.A., Fink, R., Bauer, X., Ehbauer, M., Madler,
    M. and Scriba, P.C. (1978). *GIT Labormed.* 2, 117-124.
10. Stalla, G.K., Giesemann, G., Müller, O.A., Wood, W.G.
    and Scriba, P.C. (1981). *J. Clin. Chem. Biochem.* 19,
    427-434.
11. Stalla, G.K., Hartwimmer, J. and Müller, O.A. (1984).
    Acta Endocrin.(Kbh) 105, suppl. 264,34.
12. Müller, O.A., Stalla, G.K., Hartwimmer, J., Schophol, J.
    and von Werder, K. (1984). *Acta Neurochir.* (in press).
13. Losa, M., Stalla, G.K., Müller, O.A. and von Werder, K.
    (1983). *Klin. Wschr.* 61, 1249-1253.
14. Müller, O.A., Losa, M., Oeckler, R. and von Werder, K.
    (1984). *Acta Endocrin.* (Kbh) 105, suppl. 264,33.
15. Hermus, A., Raemaekers, J.M.M., Pieters, G.F.F.M., Barte-
    link, A.K.M., Smals, A.G.H. and Kloppenborg, P.W.C.
    (1983). *Lancet* I, 776.
16. Schulte, H.M., Chrousos, G.P., Chatterji, D.C., Gold,
    P.W., Oldfield, E.H. and Loriaux, D.L. (1983). *Lancet*
    I, 1222.
17. Müller, O.A. and von Werder, K. (1983). *Endokrinologie-
    Informationen* 7, 143-146.
18. Liu, J.H., Muse, K., Contreras, P., Gibbe, D., Vale, W.,
    Rivier, J. and Yen, S.S.C. (1983). *J. Clin. Endocrinol.
    Metab.* 57, 1087-1089.
19. Rivier, C. and Vale, W. (1983). *Endocrinology* 113,939-
    942.
20. Pieters, G.F.M., Hermus, A.R.M.M., Smals, A.G.H., Barte-
    link, A.K.M., Benraad, Th.J. and Kloppenborg, P.W.C.
    (1983). *J. Clin. Endocrinol. Metab.* 57, 513-516.

PULSATILE ADMINISTRATION OF GnRH IN HYPOTHALAMIC AMENORRHEA

Gerhard Leyendecker and Ludwig Wildt

*Department of Obstetrics and Gynecology
University of Bonn
53 Bonn-Venusberg, FRG*

INTRODUCTION

Gonadotropin releasing hormone (GnRH) was the second of
the neurohumoral agents postulated by Harris more than three
decades ago to mediate hypothalamic control of anterior pituitary function that has been isolated, identified in its
structure and synthesized. Since this was achieved by the
groups of Schally and Guillemin in 1971 and the synthetic
hormone became available, GnRH has been used extensively as
a tool in neuroendocrine research. Early attempts to use this
decapeptide clinically for the treatment of reproductive disorders supposedly due to an inadequate secretion of endoge-
nousGnRH were only of limited success. Effective therapeutic
use had to await further progress in the understanding of the
physiologic significance of pulsatile gonadotropin secretion
and gonadal function. The demonstration that the pattern of
the hypophysiotropic stimulation is of critical importance
in this respect and the elucidation of the physiologic significance of pulsatile GnRH secretion have provided the ra-
tionale for the efficient use of synthetic GnRH in the treatment of GnRH deficiency.

PHYSIOLOGY AND PATHOPHYSIOLOGY

Chronic intermittent (pulsatile) administration of GnRH
as a new mode of treatment of infertility in women with hypothalamic amenorrhea is based upon the following physiological
and pathophysiological findings.

1. There is direct and indirect evidence that GnRH
   is secreted from the hypothalamus in a pulsatile
   fashion with one pulse every 60 - 90 minutes
   throughout the proliferative and periovulatory
   phase of the cycle (3,5,9,15,23,25).
2. Pulsatile stimulation of the pituitary gonadotrophs by GnRH is a prerequisite of normal pituitary gonadotrophic function (1).

Hypothalamic amenorrhea is considered to be the result of
a deficient hypothalamic secretion of GnRH (11,12). The severity of hypothalamic amenorrhea is dependent upon the degree of inpairment of hypothalamic function. On the basis of
simple clinical tests utilizing the clinical (bleeding) and
endocrine response to the administration of clomiphene,
medroxyprogesterone acetate and GnRH, respectively, a grading
system of the severity of hypothalamic amenorrhea has been
proposed (16) (Table 1).

TABLE 1

*Grading of hypothalamic amenorrhea on the basis of
clomiphene-, gestagen- and GnRH-tests.*

Grade		Results of test
1		clomiphene positive (bleeding)
2		gestagen positive (bleeding); clomiphene negative (no bleeding)
3		gestagen negative (no bleeding) with pituitary response to 100 µg of GnRH i.v..
	3a	"adult" response
	3b	"prepubertal" response
	3c	no response

Severe hypothalamic amenorrhea in women is functionally
comparable with the condition of the female rhesus monkey with
lesions on the region of the arcuate *nucleus* (18). In these
women, pulsatile administration of GnRH with an unvarying
dose and at an unchanged frequency of one pulse every 90 minutes resulted in follicular maturation, ovulation and *corpus
luteum* formation (11,12). The endocrine pattern of the normal
menstrual cycle could be completely replicated.
   Thus, it was shown that the concept of the permissive func-

tion of the hypothalamus developed in the rhesus monkey (8, 10) could be extended to the human female. These results have been confirmed by other investigators (2,4,6,7,17,19,20,21) and with the development of chronic intermittent (pulsatile) administration of GnRH by means of a small computerized pump ("Zyklomat", Ferring GmbH, Kiel, FRG) a new and practical mode of treatment of infertility in hypothalamic amenorrhea has resulted. Clinical advantage has been taken of these advances in understanding the physiology of the human menstrual cycle (13,14,16).

CLINICAL RESULTS

   Since the introduction of pulsatile administration of GnRH to women with hypothalamic amenorrhea, 115 ovulatory treatment cycles have so far been completed in our institution. Only patients with hypothalamic amenorrhea of grades 2 - 3c were included in our trial.

Dose of GnRH

   Follicular maturation and ovulation could be induced by intravenous application of 2.5 - 20 µg of GnRH per pulse in patients suffering from hypothalamic amenorrhea grades 2 - 3b, respectively. Some patients suffering from grade 3c of hypothalamic amenorrhea may require a dose of 15 - 20 µg of GnRH per pulse, while others with the same degree of severity of hypothalamic impairment ovulate with an intravenous dose of 5 µg per pulse. The different dose requirements among patients of the same grade is not clear.
   There is a dose-response relationship between the dose of GnRH administered per pulse and the effect on the ovary, as indicated by studies performed in patients with hypothalamic amenorrhea grade 3b (15,16). The mean estradiol and progesterone levels of the cycles induced with 15 - 20 µg/pulse were all above those obtained in cycles with 2.5 - 5 µg/pulse.

Substitution During the Luteal Phase

   The physiological luteotrophic hormone in the human is pituitary LH (22). In severe hypothalamic amenorrhea *corpus luteum* function immediately ceases following termination of pulsatile GnRH substitution a few days after ovulation (14). Continuation of pulsatile administration of GnRH during the whole luteal phase resulted in normal luteal function as indicated by the length of the luteal phase, the progesterone levels in serum and the number of conceptions. Previously, it was suggested to support the luteal function by one to three injections of 2500 IU of HCG once ovulation had been obtained by GnRH (13). There is, however, no indication on the basis of our data (16) that one method of luteal substitution is superior to the other in terms of pregnancy rate obtained.

Intravenous Versus Subcutaneous Application of GnRH

The same catheter used for the i.v. application of GnRH, or a butterfly needle, was used for the subcutaneous route, but without the addition of heparin to the hormone containing solution. The catheter was placed into the fat tissue of the lower abdominal wall. Ovulations could be induced with doses of 5 - 20 µg/pulse in patients with hypothalamic amenorrhea of grades 2 - 3c. Nine pregnancies were obtained with the s.c. route. However, in contrast to the i.v. application with a 100% ovulation rate, there was, over the dose range of 5 - 20 µg/pulse, an incidence of only 17 ovulatory cycles in 31 s.c. applications of GnRH. Delayed resorption of GnRH from the subcutaneous fat tissue might result in insufficient serum levels of GnRH for adequate stimulation of the pituitary gonadotrophs. It appears that for induction of ovulation via the s.c. route higher GnRH doses are required than for i.v. administration. This is in agreement with the findings of other investigators (6,17,19,21).

Ovulation- and Pregnancy-Rate

The adequate dose of GnRH provided ovulation and normal luteal function can be expected in every i.v. treatment cycle. The ovulation rate is reduced, when the s.c. route is chosen. Definitive treatment failure (no ovulation) was only observed when a false diagnosis of hypothalamic amenorrhea was made.

The pregnancy rate is remarkably high. Of 33 patients, 29 have become pregnant. Twenty four pregnancies have been completed with 29 children born, among them 3 sets of heterozygous twins and one set of triplets. Six pregnancies are still ongoing including two twin pregnancies. Eight patients aborted, one of whom had two sequential abortions probably due to active cytomegaly. Seven of these patients conceived again and had uneventful pregnancies or had a successful GnRH pregnancy before. A total of 38 conceptions were obtained in 33 patients.

The pregnancy rate, however, is critically dependent upon whether or not additional factors causing infertility of the couple are present (i.e. tubal or andrological factors).

TABLE 2

*Clinical results of pulsatile administration of GnRH
in hypothalamic amenorrhea*

33	patients
115	ovulatory treatment cycles
38	pregnancies (= 3.0 cycle per pregnancy)
8	abortions = 21%
6	multiple pregnancies = 16% (5 twins, 1 triplet)

Seventy eight ovulatory cycles were induced in 27 favourable couples in whom the hypothalamic amenorrhea constituted the only cause of infertility and 36 pregnancies were obtained (2.2 cycle per pregnancy). In summary, the pregnancy rate is comparable to that of the normal population: out of 115 ovulatory cycles obtained with exogenous GnRH 38 conceptions occurred (3.0 cycles per pregnancy) (Table 2).

Ovarian Overstimulation and Multiple Pregnancies

The feedback mechanisms of ovarian steroids of the secretion of gonadotropic hormones by the pituitary are operative during pulsatile administration of GnRH. Clinical signs of ovarian overstimulation have therefore not been observed during treatment cycles. There is, however, a dose-response relationship between the amount of GnRH administered and the ovarian response, which in turn is mediated by a dose related pituitary secretion of gonadotropins. If one considers that the recriutment of follicles, the selection of the dominant follicle and the suppression of the other accompanying follicles is dependent to a certain degree upon gonadotropic stimulation, one would expect that discrete ovarian overstimulation could cause an increased incidence of multiple pregnancies as compared to the normal population. In our study 6 multiple pregnancies were obtained with i.v. doses of 2.5 (one patient) and 5 µg/pulse (three patients), respectively. Two other multiple pregnancies were induced with i.c. and s.c. doses of 20 and 16 µg of GnRH per pulse, respectively.

CONCLUSIONS

Pulsatile administration of GnRH by means of portable pump
("Zyklomat") has proven to be an efficient and practical
method for the induction of ovulation in hypothalamic amenorrhea. The results obtained with this method of treatment are
critically dependent upon the correct selection of patients
as regards the diagnosis of hypothalamic amenorrhea. Patients
in whom this condition has previously been treated with human
gonadotropins are suitable for this mode of therapy.
In our study 38 conceptions were obtained in 33 patients.
These favourable results were obtained by a "physiological"
stimulation of the ovaries during chronic intermittent (pulsatile) administration of GnRH. On the basis of operating
negative and positive feedback mechanisms of ovarian steroids
on pituitary function occurring, the follicle itself regula-
tes the required amount of gonadotropin stimulation. However,
since there is a relationship between GnRH dose per pulse
applied and the reaction of the pituitary-ovarian axis, the
lowest efficient dose of GnRH capable of inducing ovulatory
cycles should be chosen.

ACKNOWLEDGEMENT
The skillful technical assistance of Miss Roswitha Klasen
is gratefully acknowledged.

REFERENCES

1. Belchetz, P.E., Plant, T.M., Nakai, Y., Keogh, E.J.
        and Knobil, E. (1978). *Science* 202, 631; 1979.
2. Berg, D., Mickan, H., Michael, S., Döring, K., Gloning,
        K., Jänicke, F. and Rjosk, H.K. (1983). *Arch. Gynecol.*
        233, 205.
3. Carmel, P.W., Araki, S. and Ferin, M.(1976). *Endocrinology*
        99, 243.
4. Crowley jr W.F. and McArthur, J.W. (1980). *J. Clin. Endo-
        crinol. Metab.* 51, 173.
5. Dierschke, D.J., Bhattacharya, A.N., Atkinson, L.E. and
        Knobil, E. (1970). *Endocrinology* 87, 850.
6. Hurley, D.M., Brian, R., Outch, K., Stockdale, J., Fry, A.,
        Hackman, C., Clarke, I. and Burger, H.G. (1984). *N. Engl
        J. Med.* 310, 1069.
7. Keogh, E.J., Mallal, S.A., Giles, P.F.H. and Evans, D.V.
        (1981). *Lancet* I, 147.
8. Knobil, E. (1980). *Recent Prog. Hormone Res.* 36, 53.

9.   Knobil, E. (1981). *Biol. Reprod.* 24, 44.
10. Knobil, E., Plant, T.M., Wildt, L., Belchetz, D.E. and
     Marshall, G. (1980). *Science* 207, 1371.
11. Leyendecker, G. (1979). *Eur. J. Obstet. Gynec. Reprod.
     Biol.* 9, 175.
12. Leyendecker, G., Struve, T. and Plotz, E.J. (1980). *Arch.
     Gynecol.* 229, 1371.
13. Leyendecker, G., Wildt, L. and Hansmann, M., (1980). *J.
     Clin. Endocrinol. Metab.* 51, 1214.
14. Leyendecker, G. and Wildt, L. (1981). *Therapiewoche* 31,
     6711.
15. Leyendecker, G. and Wildt, L. (1983). *In* "Neuroendocrine
     Aspects of Reproduction" (Eds R.M. Brenner, C.H.
     Phoenix, L. Norman) Academic Press, New York, p. 295.
16. Leyendecker, G. and Wildt, L. (1983). *J. Reprod. Fertil.*
     69, 397.
17. Mason, P., Adams, J., Morris, D.V., Tucker, M., Price,
     J., Voulgaris, Z., van der Spuy, Z.M., Sutherland,
     I., Chambers, G.M., White, S., Wheeler, M.J. and Jacobs,
     H.S. (1984). *Br. Med. J.* 228, 181.
18. Nakai, Y., Plant, T.M., Hess, D.K., Keogh, E.J. and Knobil,
     E. (1978). *Endocrinology* 102, 1008.
19. Reid, R.L., Leopold, G.R. and Yen, S.S.C. (1981). *Fertil.
     Steril.* 36, 553.
20. Schoemaker, J., Simons, A.H.M., Burger, C.W., Delemarred,
     H.A. and van Kessel, H. (1982). *In* "Follic. Maturation
     and Ovulation" (Eds R. Rolland, E.V. van Hall, S.G.
     Hillier, P. McNatty, J. Schoemaker) Excerpta Medica,
     Amsterdam and New York, p. 373.
21. Skarin, G., Nillius, S.J. and Wide, L.(1982). *In* "Follicu-
     lar Maturation and Ovulation" (Eds R. Rolland, E.V.
     van Hall, S.G. Hillier, P. McNatty, J. Schoemaker)
     Excerpta Medica, Amsterdam and New York, p. 398.
22. Van de Wiele, R.L., Bogumil, J., Dyrenfurth, I., Ferin,
     M., Jewelewicz, R., Warren, M., Riskhallah, T. and
     Mikhail, G. (1970). *Recent Prog. Hormone Res.* 26,
     63.
23. Van Vugt, D.A., Diefenbach, W.P. and Ferin, M. (1983). *In*
     "Programs and Abstracts", sixty-fifth Annual Meeting
     of the Endocrine Society, San Antonio, Texas; pub-
     lished by The Endocrine Society.
24. Wildt, L., Schwilden, H., Wesner, G., Roll, C., Brensing,
     K.A., Luckhaus, J., Bähr, M. and Leyendecker, G. (1983).
     In "Brain and Pituitary Peptides II. Pulsatile Ad-
     ministration of GnRH in Hypothalamic Failure: Basic
     and Clinical Aspects" (Eds G. Leyendecker, H. Stock,
     L. Wildt) Karger Verlag, Basel, p. 28.

25.   Yen, S.S.C., Tsai, C.C., Naftolin, F., van den Berg, G.
      and Ajabar, L. (1972). *J. Clin. Endocrinol. Metab.*
      <u>34</u>, 671.

ADVANCES IN SOMATOSTATIN RESEARCH

A. Gómez-Pan*, M.D. Rodriguez-Arnao[+] and E. del Pozo[++]

*Endocrinology Department, C.N.E.Q., Pabellon 8, Faculty of Medicine, 28040 Madrid, Spain

+Endocrinology Service, Hospital Provincial, 28009 Madrid, Spain

++Experimental Therapeutics Department, SANDOZ LTD., 4002 Basel, Switzerland

INTRODUCTION

During the past decade, since the isolation, characterization and synthesis of somatostatin (SS-14)(1,2), it has been firmly established that SS-14 possesses powerful antisecretory activity on both endocrine and exocrine functions (3-5). SS-14 has proven to be a valuable research tool for investigating various physiological events, particularly at the pituitary and gastroenteropancreatic level. Nevertheless, its therapeutic potential, which is realized only in acute or subacute situations, has been limited because of its variety of effects, the need of intravenous administration and its extremely short life in circulation. These limitations prompted the search for structural analogues or other naturally occurring molecules which would exhibit prolonged activity and more selectivity in their effects. We shall review recent developments in the area of somatostatin research with special emphasis on the clinical applications of new derivatives.

NATURALLY OCCURRING SOMATOSTATINS

Somatostatin-28

Several larger molecular forms of SS-14 have ben extracted from brain and peripheral tissues. One of these forms has been isolated from porcine intestine (6) and *hypothalamus* (7), and

DOPAMINE AND NEUROENDOCRINE ACTIVE SUBSTANCES
ISBN 0 12 209045 4

from ovine *hypothalamus* (8). Its structure was shown to be
an amino-terminally extended form comprising 28 aminoacids
(9-12). It was subsequently synthetysed. We have previously reported a comparative study describing the effects of
SS-14 and Somatostatin 28 (SS-28) on the growth hormone and
prolactin response to arginine in humans (13). In this paper
we deal with the effects of SS-28 on anterior pituitary and
pancreatic endocrine secretion in healthy men and in patients
with acromegaly and primary hypothyroidism.

Effect of SS-28 on anterior pituitary hormones. Five normal
subjects undertook a standard arginine stimulation test 30
minutes after the beginning of a two hour infusion of either
saline, SS-14 (62.5 mcg/hr) or SS-28 (125 mcg/hr). The GH
response to arginine was partially inhibited by SS-14 and
completely abolished by equimolar doses of SS-28 (Fig. 1).

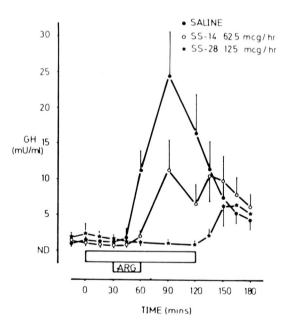

*Fig. 1. Effect of somatostatin-14 and somatostatin-28 on
arginine-induced growth hormone release.*

In addition to its greater GH inhibitory potency, SS-28 also caused a 30-minute delay in the appearance of the rebound after the infusion was discontinuated. These data confirm and extend our previous report (13) and also the data of Millar and coworkers (14) who evaluated the relative GH inhibitory potency of SS-14 and SS-28 in response to insulin-induced hypoglycaemia. Four acromegalic patients received a 60 minute-infusion of either saline, SS-14 (125 mcg/hr) or SS-28 (250 mcg/hr). The reduction of GH levels in response to both forms was similar. However, return to baseline values occurred 10 minutes after cessation of the SS-14 infusion and only 45 minutes after discontinuing SS-28 administration (Fig. 2)(15).

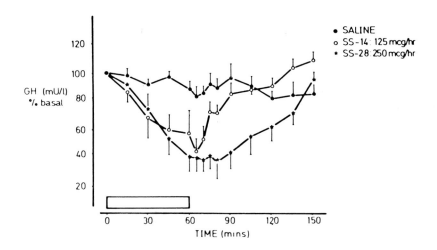

Fig. 2. Effects of somatostatin-14 and somatostatin-28 on growth hormone levels in patients with acromegaly.

Both SS-14 and SS-28 reduced the TSH response to thyrotropin-releasing hormone (TRH) in normal subjects, but their inhibitory potency appeared to be equal (Fig. 3).

Similarly, the elevated TSH levels observed in six patients with primary hypothyriodism were identically suppressed by SS-14 of SS-28. (Fig. 4). Neither SS-14 nor SS-28 had any effect on both basal, TRH-, arginine- or hypoglycaemia-induced prolactin hypersecretion. The release of ACTH, as assessed by the cortisol response to insulin-induced hypoglycaemia, was not affected by SS-14 or SS-28 in normal individ-

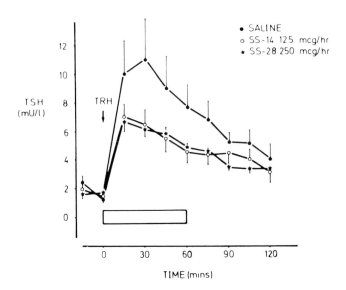

Fig. 3. Effects of somatostatin-14 and somatostatin-28 on thyrotropin-releasing hormone - mediated thyrotropin release in man.

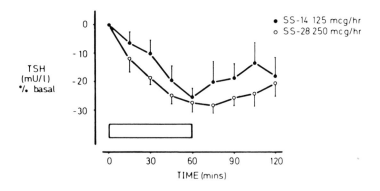

Fig. 4. Effects of somatostatin-14 and somatostatin-28 on basal thyrotropin levels in patients with primary hypothyroidism.

uals. We have not observed any effect of SS-14 or SS-28 on basal gonadotropin levels. However, Millar *et al.* (16) have reported that SS-28 blocked the gonadotropin response to gonadotropin-releasing hormone. The explanation of this effect, which is not shared by the tetradecapeptide, is not known.

Effect of SS-28 on pancreatic hormones. The insulin-response to a standard arginine stimulation test was blunted by SS-14 and completely abolished by equimolar concentrations of SS-28 (Fig. 5). However, the insulin release elicited by a protein rich meal was more powerfully inhibited by SS-28 than by SS-14 (17). Both peptides reduced basal glucagon blood levels and partially inhibited its response to arginine (Fig. 6) or to a protein rich meal (17). Both molecular forms exhibited the same inhibitory power as far as glucagon is concerned.

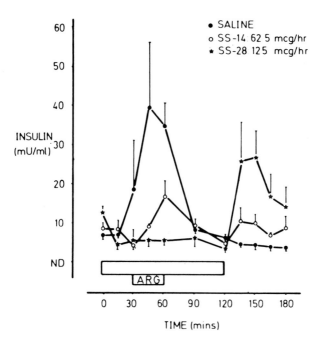

Fig. 5. Effects of somatostatin-14 and somatostatin-28 on arginine-induced insulin release.

We have previously shown that both SS-14 and SS-28 are capable of inhibiting the pancreatic polypeptide response to a protein rich meal (17). On an equimolar basis, the inhibitory potency of both molecular forms appears to be similar. Nevertheless, the effect of SS-28 is longer lasting than that of SS-14 (18).

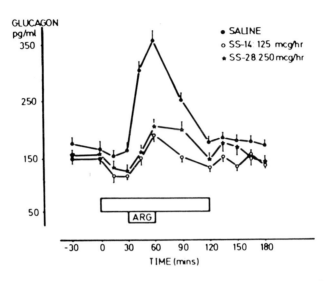

Fig. 6. Effects of somatostatin-14 and somatostatin-28 on arginine-induced glucagon release.

SOMATOSTATIN ANALOGUES

    In order to circumvent the drawbacks of the therapeutic
potential of the naturally occurring forms of SS-14, a large
number of structural analogues have been synthesized (19-22).
These were designed to obtain enhanced, prolonged an more selective activities. In addition, they provide a useful tool
for structure-function relationship studies. It has been established that the terminal carboxy group is not required for biological activity (23,24). Likewise, alterations at the N-terminus do not alter the potency of the molecule (25). Early
structure-activity studies were designed using the strategy
of systematic replacement of each aminoacid by L-Alanine,
thereby identifying the "active core" of the peptide (21).
Thus it was found that residues Gly[2], Asn[5], Thr[10], Thr[12] and
Ser[13] do not contribute substantially to the activity of the
peptide. However, the hydrophobic aminoacids Phe[6], Phe[7], Trp[8]
and Lys[9] are involved in receptor binding and activation,
forming the essential pharmacophore of the SS-14 molecule
(22,25). The residue Thr[10] is an essential spacer and tne two
cysteins plus the other aminoacids contribute to the proper
three-dimensional structure of the four critical residues (22).
A cyclic structure is required for receptor activation. The
reported full activity of a reduced linear form of the peptide

is likely to be due to spontaneous oxidation to the cyclized, native form under the experimental conditions (25).

It has been shown that brain extracts cleave SS-14 at the Trp^8-Lys^9 bond (26). Thus, replacement of the residue Trp^8 by its dextroisomer prevents its endogenous degradation and makes the molecule six to eight times more potent (27). Stepwise modification of the SS-14 active fragment led to the synthesis of a number of oligo-peptides which retained full activity. Some of these conformationally stabilized analogues have been shown to be active when administered by several routes, including the oral, to be longer acting and to possess a certain degree of inhibitory selectivity (28-30).

SMS 201-995: A new Octapeptide Analogue

Bauer and coworkers (31) synthesized a cyclic octapeptide analogue which was named selective minisomatostatin (SMS 201-995 Sandoz)(Fig. 7).

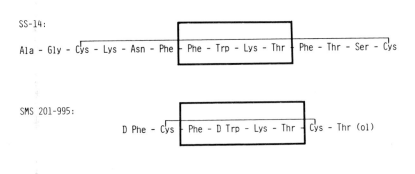

SS-14:

Ala - Gly - Cys - Lys - Asn - Phe - Phe - Trp - Lys - Thr - Phe - Thr - Ser - Cys

SMS 201-995:

D Phe - Cys - Phe - D Trp - Lys - Thr - Cys - Thr (ol)

Fig. 7. Biochemical structures of native somatostatin (SS) and the low molecular analogue SMS 201-995.

As can be deducted, the structure of SMS 201-995 mimics the essential pharmacophore of the native SS molecule: the active residues $Phe^7-Trp^8-Lys^9$ are kept in position, with a dextroisomer replacing Trp^8 which enhances resistance to degradation. The essential Thr^{10} is also maintained, and the structure is completed by a disulphide bridge between two cysteins. The aromatic side chain, at the N-terminus, (D-Phe), can occupy the conformational space of the essential residue Phe^6 in the native

SS peptide, and also protects the Cys-Cys bridge. The side chain of the amino-alcohol Thr-ol at the C-terminus represents Thr^{12} in the native molecule and protects against enzymatic degradation. Early pharmacodynamic studies conducted by Bauer *et al.* (31) have shown that SMS 201-995 is active when administered intravenously, intramuscularly, subcutaneously or orally to the experimental animal. It has also been shown that this derivative is highly resistant to degradation by enzyme mixtures or by kidney homogenates. In comparative *in vivo* studies (rat), SMS 201-995 was 70 times more potent than GH inhibitor and longer lasting than SS-14. Bauer and his colleagues have also shown this peptide to possess a certain degree of specificity. Thus, in the rat, it is 22 times more GH/insulin selective and 3 times more GH/glucagon selective when compared to native somatostatin. Comparative studies in the rhesus monkey have shown that SMS 201-995 is 45 times more effective than SS-14 to inhibit GH secretion, 11 times more active to suppress glucagon and only 1.3 more active to inhibit insulin release (31). Toxicological assessment has revealed that SMS 201-995 is well tolerated by both laboratory animals and man, and devoid of unwanted side effects (32), suggesting that this peptide is suitable for clinical studies.

Pharmacokinetics of SMS 201-995. Plasma levels of administered SMS 201-995 have been measured by specific radioimmunoassay in normal subjects. During an intravenous infusion, plasma SMS 201-995 levels rise in a dose-dependent fashion, to reach a plateau 90 minutes after the onset of the infusion. The elimination half-life was 41-58 min (32). After subcutaneous administration, plasma levels peaked at 15-30 min after injection. The elimination half-life was 113 min (Fig. 8). Intravenously administered SMS 201-995 gave 6-30 times higher plasma levels and was eliminated about 10 times slower than an equimolar dosis of the native peptide. These findings encouraged the further development of this derivative for clinical use. Results obtained from studies conducted in normal volunteers and in patients are presented below.

Hormonal profile of SMS 201-995. In normal subjects this peptide was found to inhibit GH and glucagon elevations induced by biological *stimuli* such as sleep, protein intake or exercise in doses of 10 mcg/h i.v. or 50-100 mcg s.c. (33). GH reductions of 75 to 89% were observed at these dosage strengths. A simultaneous fall in plasma insulin was also recorded. However, in another series of tests in which arginine was applied at different time intervals, asynchronous GH and insulin effects were observed. Thus, an arginine infusion administered three hours after injection of SMS 201-995 was unable to elicit

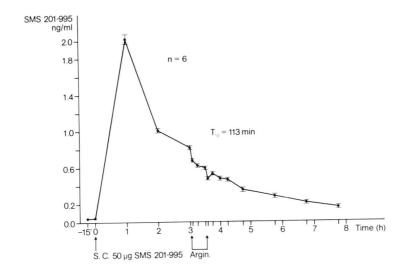

Fig. 8. Plasma kinetics of SMS 201-995 after subcutaneous administration.

a GH peak whereas insulin exhibited a normal response (32). These findings may have clinical relevance since hyperglycaemia can be prevented by timely administration of the peptide. In general, the GH secretory rebound commonly seen after stopping SS-14 is missing after SMS 201-995 administration. This was interpreted as reflecting a prolonged action probably maintained by its high potency and slow plasma clearance (33), (Fig. 9).

Screening of the effect of SMS 201-995 on other gastro-intestinal hormones has revealed a broad spectrum of inhibitory actions typical of somatostatin. A detailed report has been published elsewhere (34).

Plewe and coworkers (35) have recently reported that the subcutaneous administration of 50 mcg of SMS 201-995 was followed by a reduction of circulating GH levels to normal values in six out of seven patients with active acromegaly (Fig. 10). Their results have been corroborated by other investigators (36, 37,38). The reduction in GH levels induced by SMS 201-995 in patients with acromegaly is long lasting, being suppressed for up to nine hours after subcutaneous administration. When ad-

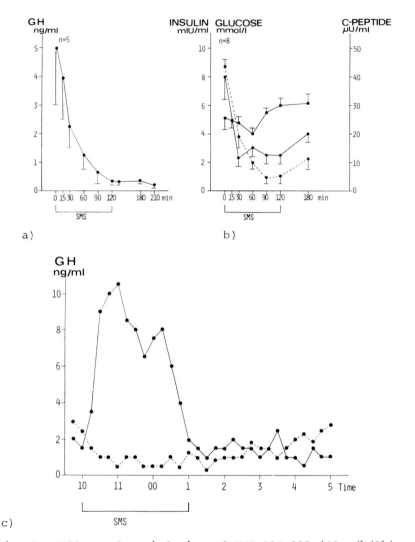

a)

b)

c)

Fig. 9a. Effect of an infusion of SMS 201-995 (10ug/h/2h) on basal plasma GH. There is a gradual decline in GH levels to subnormal values. Absence of rebound phenomenon is conspicuous.

Fig. 9b. Under SMS 201-995 (10ug/h/2h) plasma insulin and C-peptide descend in a parallel manner whereas glucose adopts a characteristic biphasic pattern.(C-peptide dotted line).

Fig. 9c. Effect of an infusion of SMS 201-995 (10ug/h/5h) during sleep in a normal subject. The GH peak is completely suppressed. Again, a rebound effect is missing.

ministered with appropriate anticipation to meals *(vide infra)*,
SMS 201-995 is a selective GH inhibitory peptide, having negligible effects on other pituitary or enteropancreatic secre-
tions. SMS 201-995 may well represent the GH-selective somatostatin analogue, suitable for the medical management of patients with acromegaly. Long term clinical trials are now in
progress, and preliminary data suggest that 50 to 100 mcg
b.i.d. or t.i.d. subcutaneously effectively suppresses GH levels and improves the clinical manifestations of the disease
dramatically (39).

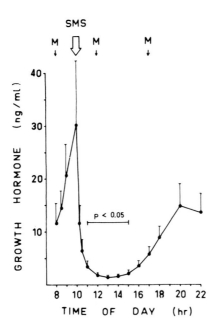

*Fig. 10. Effect of a single subcutaneous injection of 50 ug
SMS 201-995 on plasma GH in 7 acromegalic subjects.*

There have been recent reports on the favorable effect of
SMS 201-995 in the management of endocrine active gastrointestinal tumors (40,41). Furthermore, a dampening effect on
insulin hypersensitivity has been reported in brittle dia-
betics (42). As a result, a substantial reduction in daily
insulin requirements was recorded. Fig. 11 depicts the hormone profile of such a patient receiving subcutaneous injections of 100 and 50 mcg SMS 201-995 before breakfast and
dinner respectively. There is a clear reduction in plasma GH
and glucagon levels following administration of the peptide,

and glucose increments following meals are considerably reduced. The insulin dose in the evening is reduced by 50% in
order to prevent possible hypoglycemic episodes during sleep.
Inhibition of GH secretion with subcutaneous SMS 201-995
during night sleep may prove effective in counteracting the
so called "dawn phenomenon". This consists of frank or near
hypoglycemic episodes about 2-3 a.m. followed by a progressive
rise in blood glucose to reach highest values around breakfast time. Recent investigations have shown GH to play an
important role in the generation of this phenomenon.

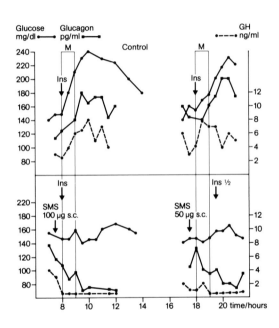

*Fig. 11. Effect of 100 and 50 ug SMS 201-995 administered
subcutaneously on plasma glucose, GH and glucagon, in a diabetic individual (Type I). The glucose increment following
a standard meal (M) is flattened after injection of SMS 201-
995. This effect is concomitant with a substantial fall in
circulating GH and glucagon.*

Other Long-Acting Somatostatin Analogues

In 1977, Brown and coworkers (43) reported on a potent decapeptide with the code name CVY-41,747. This substance exerted
a predominant and long-acting inhibitory action on glucagon

and GH secretion in the experimental animal (44). In diabetic patients, a subcutaneous infusion at the relatively high dose of 10-50 mcg/kg administered during 30 minutes in combination with insulin effectively limited postprandial hyperglycaemia and reduced glucagon and plasma triglycerides for 120 to 300 minutes respectively (45). Other derivatives have now entered clinical evaluation but information at the present time is too scanty to allow a precise evaluation.

CONCLUSIONS

In summary, SS-28 appears to be more potent than its congener SS in the inhibition of GH and insulin secretion, and its effects on GH are longer lasting. Both molecular forms are equipotent in the suppression of TSH and glucagon release. Neither SS nor SS-28 have any effect on PRL, ACTH or gonadotrophin secretion.

The reported differences in the inhibitory power of SS and SS-28, their different tissue concentration and their distinct receptor binding activity strongly argue in favour that SS-28 is not a mere precursor of SS tetradecapeptide, but has an independent physiological function. Though more potent than SS in suppressing GH and insulin secretion, SS-28 retains the multiple effects of SS and has also a short half life (6.1 min.), which reduces considerably its therapeutic expectations. On the base of its high potency and prolonged action, the new somatostatin analogue SMS 201-995 represents a useful tool in the investigation of growth hormone disorders and diabetes. Preliminary results of acute studies justify its full evaluation on chronic administration.

ACKNOWLEDGEMENTS

The comparative studies with somatostatin-14 and somatostatin-28 were carried out in collaboration with Dres G.M. Besser and J.A.H. Wass (London), R. Hall (Cardiff) and A.V. Schally, D.H. Coy and A.M. Comaru-Schally (New Orleans). We wish also to thank the excellent technical help of Mr. J.R. Arnao.

Part of the data discussed here were obtained thanks to the support of the Fondo de Investigaciones Sanitarias del Insalud, Spain (Grant 83/0713).

REFERENCES

1. Brazeau, P., Vale, W., Burgus, R., Ling, N., Butcher, M., Rivier, J. and Guillemin, R. (1973). *Science* 179, 77-79.
2. Coy, D.H., Coy, E.J., Arimura, A. and Schally, A.V. (1973). *Biochem. Biophys. Res. Commun.* 54, 1267-1273.
3. Gómez-Pan, A. and Hall, R. (1977). *Clin. Endocrinol. Metab.* 6, 181-200.
4. Gómez-Pan, A. and Rodriguez-Arnao, M.D. (1983). *Clin. Endocrinol. Metab.* 12, 469-507.
5. Reichlin, S. (1983). *N. Engl. Med.* 309, 1495-1501, and 309, 1556-1563.
6. Pradayrol, L. Chayvialle, J.A., Carlquist, M. and Mutt, V. (1978). *Biochem. Biophys.Res. Commun.* 85, 701-708.
7. Schally, A.V., Huang, W.Y., Chang, R.R.C., Arimura, A., Redding, T.W., Millar, R.P., Hunkapiller, M.W. and Hood, L.E. (1980). *Proc. Natl. Acad. Sci.* 77, 4489-4493.
8. Bohlen, P., Brazeau, P., Benoit, R., Ling, N., Esch, F. and Guillemin, R. (1980). *Biochem. Biophys. Res. Commun.* 96, 725-734.
9. Esch, F., Bohlen, P., Ling, N., Benoit, R., Brazeau, P. and Guillemin, R. (1980). *Proc. Natl. Acad. Sci.* 77, 6827-6831.
10. Ling, N., Esch, F., Davis, D., Mercado, M., Regno, M., Bohlen, P., Brazeau, P. and Guillemin, R. (1980). *Biochem. Biophys. Res. Commun.* 95, 945-951.
11. Meyers, C.A., Murphy, W.A., Redding, R.W., Coy, D.H. and Schally, A. (1980). *Proc. Natl. Acad. Sci.* 77, 6171-6174.
12. Brazeau, P., Ling, N., Esch, F., Bohlen, P,, Benoit, R. and Guillemin, R. (1981). *Reg. Pept.* 1, 255-264.
13. Rodriguez-Arnao, M.D., Gómez-Pan, A., Rainbow, S.J., Woodhead, S., Comaru-Schally, A.M., Schally, A.V., Meyers, C.A., Coy, D.H. and Hall, R. (1981). *Lancet* i, 353-356.
14. Millar, R.P., Klaff, L.J., Barron, J.L., Levitt, N.S. and Ling, N. (1983). *Clin. Endocrinol.* 18, 277-285.
15. Rodriguez-Arnao, M.D., Wass, J.A.H., Webb, S., Gómez-Pan, A., Rainbow, S.J., Woodhead, F., Owens, D.R., Besser, G.M., Coy, D.H., Comaru-Schally, A.M., Schally, A.V. and Hall, R. (1984). *In* "Somatostatin" (Ed. S. Raptis), pp. 312-313. Tübinger Chronik.
16. Millar, R.P., Klaff, L.J., Barron, J., Levitt, N.S. and Ling, N. (1982). *Clin. Endocrinol.* 17, 103-107.

17. Marco, J., Correas, I., Zulueta, M.A., Vincent, E., Coy, D.H., Comaru-Schally, A.M., Schally, A.V., Rodriguez-Arnao, M.D. and Gómez-Pan, A. (1983). *Horm. Metab. Res.* 15, 363-366.
18. Srikant, C.B. and Patel, Y.C. (1981). *Nature* 294, 259-260.
19. Brown, M.P., Coy, D.H., Gómez-Pan, A., Hirst, B.H., Hunter, M., Meyers, C., Reed, J.D., Schally, A.V. and Shaw, B. (1978). *J. Physiol.* 277, 1-14.
20. Meyers, C.A. and Coy, D.H. (1980). *In* "Gastrointestinal Hormones" (Ed. G.B.J. Glass), pp. 363-386. Raven Press, New York.
21. Rivier, J., Brown, M., Rivier, C., Ling, N. and Vale, W. (1977). *In* "Peptides 1976" (Ed. A. Loffet), pp. 427-451. Editions de l'Université de Bruxelles, Brussels.
22. Vale, W., Rivier, J., Ling, N. and Brown, M. (1978). *Metabolism* 27, (suppl. 1), 1391-1401.
23. Sarantakis, D., McKinley, W.A. and Grant, N.H. (1973). *Biochem. Biophys. Res. Commun.* 55, 538-542.
24. Veber, D.F., Stracham, R.C., Bergstrand, S.J., Holly, F.W., Homnick, C.F. and Hirschmann, R. (1976). *J. Amer. Chem. Soc.* 98, 2367-2369.
25. Schonbrunn, A., Rorstad, O.P., Westendorf, J.M. and Martin, J.B. (1983). *Endocrinology* 113, 1559-1567.
26. Marks, N. and Stern, F. (1975). *FEBS Lett.* 55, 220-224.
27. Rivier, J., Brown, M. and Vale, W. (1975). *Biochem. Biophys. Res. Commun.* 65, 746-751.
28. Murphy, W.A., Meyers, C.A. and Coy, D.H. (1981). *Endocrinology* 109, 491-495.
29. Veber, D.F., Holly, F.W., Nutt, R.F., Bergstrand, S.J., Brady, S.F., Hirschmann, R., Glitzer, M.S. and Saperstein, R. (1979). *Nature* 280, 512-514.
30. Veber, D.F., Saperstein, R., Nutt, R.F., Freidinger, R.M., Brady, S.F., Curley, P., Perlow, D.S., Paleveda, W.J., Colton, C.D., Zacchei, A.G., Tocco, D.J., Hoff, D.R., Vandlen, R.L., Gerich, J.E., Hall, L., Mandarino, L., Cordes, E.H., Anderson, P.S. and Hirschmann, R. (1984). *Life Sci.* 34, 1371-1378.
31. Bauer, W., Briner, V., Doepfner, W., Haller, R., Huguenin, R., Marbach, P., Petcher, T.J. and Pless, J. (1982). *Life Sci.* 31, 1133-1140.
32. del Pozo, E., Schlüter, K., Neufeld, M., Tortosa, F., Wendel, L. and Kerp, L. *Acta Endocrinol.* (in press).
33. Marbach, P., Neufeld, M. and Pless, J. (1985). *In* "Somatostatin" (Eds Y.C. Patel and G.S. Tannenbaum), Plenum Press, New York (in press).
34. Kraenzlin, M., Wood, S., Neufeld, M., Adrian, T. and Bloom, S.R. *Experientia* (in press).

35. Plewe, G., Beyer, J., Krause, U., Neufeld, M. and del
    Pozo, E. (1984). *Lancet* 2, 782-784.
36. Ch'ng, L.J.C., Sandler, L.M., Kraenzlin, M.E., Burrin, J.M.,
    Joplin, G.F. and Bloom, S.R. (1985). *Brit. Med. J.*
    290, 284-285.
37. Althoff, P.H., Böttger, B., Rosak, C., Neufeld, M., Knigge,
    H., Jungmann, E., Lacey, F. and Schöffling, K. (1984).
    In "7th International Congress of Endocrinology", p.
    324. Excerpta Medica, Intern. Congress Series 652,
    Amsterdam, The Netherlands.
38. Lamberts, S.W.J., Oosterom, R., Neufeld, M. and del Pozo,
    E. (1985). *J. Clin. Endocrinol. Metab.* (in press).
39. Lamberts, S.W.J., Uitterlinden, P., Verschoor, L., van
    Dongen, K.J. and del Pozo, E. *New Eng. J. Med.* (in
    press).
40. Kraenzlin, M., Ch'ng, L.J.C., Wood, S.M. and Bloom, S.R.
    (1984). *Gut* 25, A 576.
41. von Werder, K., Losa, M., Müller, O.A., Schweiberer, L.,
    Fahlbusch, R. and del Pozo, E. (1984). *Lancet* 2, 282-
    283.
42. Plewe, G., Noelken, G., Krause, U., Kuestner, E., Kahaly,
    G., del Pozo, E. and Beyer, J. (submitted).
43. Brown, M., Rivier, J. and Vale, W. (1977). *Science* 196,
    1467-1469.
44. Lien, E. and Sarantakis, D. (1979). *Diabetologia* 17, 59-
    64.
45. Dimitriadis, G., Tessari, P. and Gerich, J. (1983).
    Metabolism 32, 987-992.

Index